SPIRITUAL AWAKENING ACADEMY

KUNDALINI AWAKENING

I0145941

Mind Power Through Chakra Meditation, and Yoga.

Empath healing for Beginners, Psychic Abilities, Intuition, Astral Travel, Mindfulness, Overcome Insomnia, Anxiety & Depression

*By **Spiritual Awakening Academy***

Table of Contents

INTRODUCTION **3**

CHAPTER 1: KUNDALINI BASICS **5**

CHAPTER 2: THE BASICS OF MEDITATION **13**

CHAPTER 3: THE ENERGY OF PRANA **32**

CHAPTER 4: PSYCHIC ABILITIES **64**

CHAPTER 5: PSYCHIC SKILLS **82**

CHAPTER 6: CLAIRVOYANCE & OTHER PSYCHIC GIFTS **108**

CHAPTER 7: ASTRAL TRAVEL **113**

CHAPTER 8: HOW TO AWAKEN KUNDALINI **126**

CHAPTER 9: TERMINOLOGIES **134**

CONCLUSION **139**

Introduction

Kundalini awakening journeys are life-changing. Once you start, you will never look at life the same. Even if you were to begin the awakening process and then restrict it and let your Kundalini go dormant again, you could expect to be forever changed. The energy is *that* powerful. Fortunately for you, almost no one looks back after their awakening. The energy is pure, addicting, empowering, and so full of love and joy that it truly is unlike anything you have ever experienced before.

The best way to get the most out of this book is to ensure that you read it cover to cover first, then use it as a reference guide as needed. "*Kundalini Awakening*" is written with the intention of guiding you through all of the stages of awakening and supporting you in beginning your own daily Kundalini practice that you can use for life. This book is structured in a way that supports you in having all of the knowledge you need to begin your awakening. It is important that you start with the knowledge section first, as this will enable you to understand exactly what it is that you are awakening and what you can expect from the process. Then, you can proceed to move into the actual practices that contribute to the awakening.

As you go through your Kundalini journey, you may find times where you need more support in your awakening. Natural stages in your cycle may lead to you feeling particularly low on energy, closed, restricted, or otherwise struggling to maintain a healthy, balanced flow. During those times, referring back to this guide can support you in getting back to the basics and clearing out your channels so that you can resume your balanced Kundalini flow.

Realize that this journey is different for everyone. While the foundations are the same and there are many synchronicities between those who are awakening, you will likely become aware of the fact that some of the information you read or pick up along the way seems irrelevant to you. This is natural. Stay in a state of flow and allow yourself to continue moving through. As you will learn in this book, allowing and accepting are the easiest ways to keep yourself in a state of Kundalini flow.

Chapter 1: Kundalini Basics

The Kundalini, also known as *goddess power* or *serpent power*, is said to possess immense power. It is located at the base of the spine. The practice of awakening the Kundalini is very much known in India, but it is also being practiced in different parts of the world. The Kundalini is said to look like a coiled serpent at the base of the spine. Once awakened, it becomes a gateway or a key to great psychic powers, and even enlightenment.

Why is it important to learn/practice Kundalini?

It is important to learn and practice Kundalini awakening because it can take you to a higher spiritual level. It is not uncommon for people to suddenly be stuck in a plateau in their spiritual life. It is a state where there seems to be no more progress or development. During this stage, awakening the Kundalini is often one of the best things to do.

Of course, you do not need to be in a spiritual plateau before you learn and practice to awaken the Kundalini. In fact, this is something that you can do at any time. If you want to go deeper into spirituality, if you want to be able to harness psychic powers, then this is the one for you. However, it should be noted that acquiring psychic powers is not the primary goal of Kundalini awakening. The acquisition of such powers is merely incidental to the process of Kundalini awakening.

The differences between Kundalini and Prana

Some people confuse Kundalini and prana with each other. It should be noted that these two terms are related to each other, but they are not the same. Prana is the pervading energy that exists inside you and all around you. When the Kundalini is awakened, a strong rush of prana surges through the body. Take note that Kundalini and prana are different from each other.

However, in some sense, it can be said that Kundalini is also prana. This is because of the belief that literally everything is made of prana. However, technically speaking, they are not the same, just as a chakra is different from Prana.

The Kundalini is often awakened by drawing more prana into the location where the Kundalini resides, which is at the base of the spine. Clearly, they are not the same.

The relationship between Kundalini and Chi

Chi is another term for prana. Prana is referred to by different terms depending on the culture or location. In China, prana is called as chi. In Greece, it is referred to as pneuma. In ancient Polynesia, prana was called mana. The term prana is a term that is used in India. Still, all these terms refer to the same energy.

The health benefits of Kundalini

The awakening of the Kundalini has been linked to various health benefits. It promotes good health at many levels. It regulates and corrects blood pressure; it is also an effective stress reliever; it can fight and even cure diabetes and other diseases, as well as a host of many other physical benefits. This also involves relief from stomach and liver problems, even issues with kidney stones and gallstones. There are even those who claim that awakening the Kundalini can cure serious diseases like cancer. Indeed, when you experience the power that surges through your body upon awakening of the Kundalini, you will know that indeed, everything is possible. Having clarity of thought is a very common benefit of awakening the Kundalini, as well as increased focus, attention, and mental power.

It is also worth noting that many of these benefits can be enjoyed even without fully awakening your Kundalini. The different practices themselves, as you will learn from this book, can give you tons of health benefits. Of course, if you want to experience the benefits to their fullest potential, then you need to actually awaken your Kundalini.

Different Kundalini exercises and meditations

It should be noted that there is no single exercise or meditation technique that will guarantee the awakening of the Kundalini. The accumulative spiritual practices and spiritual maturity are needed for this to happen. All the practices in this book will help you awaken your Kundalini. However, be reminded that gaining knowledge is not enough. You also need to put that knowledge into actual and continuous practice.

You may wonder why this book is full of mental and meditative techniques. The reason is that the awakening the Kundalini is more of a mental effort and practice. You should expect to engage in long hours of meditation. However, there are also physical exercises that can help you awaken the Kundalini. After all, physical exercises of any kind are a natural way of cleansing the body of negative energies. Depending on your physical fitness, you may engage in a physical activity or exercise of your choice. For starters, you might want to engage in some walking exercises. If you are a feeling fit and healthy, then you can go for a jog or a good run. Needless to say, exercising is also good for the physical body.

The best way to awaken the Kundalini is by doing meditation. As you read this book, you will learn different meditation techniques. Some of these meditation techniques will directly empower and engage your Kundalini, while others may do so indirectly. Still, it is worth noting that all meditation practices help in awakening the Kundalini. Hence, you can rest for sure that no effort will ever be wasted.

The effects of Kundalini activation on the body, emotions, and the mind

As to the emotions, it will make you feel more centered and calm. In fact, even before you reach the stage of awakening, you will already enjoy its positive effects on the emotional level. You will feel less stressed, and you will be more in control of yourself and your emotions.

With regard to the mind, you will have more mental clarity. You will be able to think and analyze things more clearly. It will give you such clarity that you have never experienced in your life. In fact, it is with such mental clarity that is tantamount to having complete peace of mind.

How Kundalini feels

If your Kundalini is still dormant, then you might not feel it at all. However, the more that you work on your Kundalini, the more that you can feel it, especially when you do the meditation techniques that directly engage the Kundalini. At the moment of the awakening of the Kundalini, you can expect for a powerful rush of energy through your body.

This happens as the energy is released and the serpentine power shoots up through the other chakras. The feeling is often reported to be warm as energy is usually warm. It is also a pleasurable release. Some even say that it is more pleasurable than having an orgasm. It is, you can say, some form of spiritual bliss.

How to clear the blockages that prevent Kundalini from rising smoothly

Blockages can prevent the awakening and rising of the Kundalini. In order to avoid this from happening, you need to ensure that there is a free flow of energy through the energy channels meridians. You should also ensure that your chakras are cleansed and aligned.

However, what causes these blockages? There are many causes of blockages. A common cause of this is having too much stress. In the modern world, being stressed has become very common; and this is actually a sad thing, as it means that many people do not enjoy a free flow of energy. If you want to activate your Kundalini, then you need to be sure to manage your stress levels effectively. It should be noted that stress itself is not bad; it is when you fail to manage it properly that it becomes bad for you. There are many other causes that can impede the free flow of energy, such as having bad experiences, emotional breakdown, psychic attacks, and others. When treating blockages, it is important to note the reason or the main cause of the problem. A common mistake is to treat a blockage without attending to what causes it in the first place. Therefore, if a blockage is due to your stress at work, then you need to make some adjustments at work. You cannot just treat the effect or the result without going after the source.

Therefore, removing of any blockages or healing should be done on two levels, physical and spiritual.

On the physical level, you may have to make some lifestyle changes.

Chapter 2: The Basics of Meditation

Meditation is strongly related to mystical experiences and Kundalini syndromes. According to a study, it is more effective than yoga and prayer in creating Kundalini syndromes. It is possible that this is because meditation involves an inner focus, which is not always involved in yoga or prayer. After all, meditation goes beyond a particular religious belief or practice, and it is something that is shared by varying cultures throughout history.

Because regular meditators experience Kundalini more often, it may mean that it is caused by the meditations or because dedicated meditators are predisposed for Kundalini experiences. No matter what the case may be, you will benefit if you regularly meditate. Not only will you train your mind to make it more capable of directing and withstanding energy, you will also receive perks like improved moods, self-control and overall health.

Mystical traditions assert that meditating upon a deity, a guru, a holy man/woman or a sacred concept will make you acquire their energetic qualities. This can mean gazing at a picture of them, chanting their name or mantra, imagining them, or emotionally connecting to them. There are certain gurus who are said to convey Shaktipat to their disciples by letting them connect to their energy via meditation.

Transcendental Meditation may activate the Kundalini – some of those who practice TM have experienced the Kundalini syndrome. This involves meditation with a mantra that may be given by the guru. An often-used mantra is "ong namo guru dev namo" which is translated to "I bow to the divine within." This connects your energy to a line of enlightened masters, ensuring that the wisdom you receive is reliable and the energy controlled.

Meditation and Multiple Practices

Based on research on meditators and Kundalini experiencers, meditation and multiple transpersonal practices increase the chances of Kundalini awakening.

It was discovered that the total amount of practice is more important than the frequency, pattern, and social conditions of practicing. This means that it's good if you meditate a lot of times so the effect will accumulate.

Prayer

Prayer leads to mystical experiences when there are positive emotions like adoration and gratitude. When prayer involves requests or confession of sins, or if it is done out of obligation, mystical experiences occur less frequently. When praying, include in your intention that you want to be closer to God or to your idea of the Divine. You may ask that this happen specifically via Kundalini awakening, but sometimes it may occur in another form. Catholics or Christians may experience the descent of the Holy Spirit – it is similar to the Kundalini but in a form that their belief systems are already predisposed to accept.

Yoga

There are many kinds of yoga; some deal specifically with Kundalini activation. Regardless of whether yoga is done for Kundalini or not, Kundalini will more likely be awakened if yoga is practiced contemplatively. In contrast, if yoga is done mechanically and treated only as a means to attain fitness, Kundalini will remain dormant.

Yoga generally deals with physical exercises (asanas and mudras), chanting (mantras), breath control (pranayama), meditation, concentration, and visualization.

Some forms of yoga that deal with Kundalini are the following:

- Kundalini yoga/Laya yoga: Kundalini yoga incorporates Hatha yoga, Kriya yoga, visualization and meditation.

- Hatha yoga: There are particular Hatha yoga practices that are said to raise Kundalini such as mula bandha, jalandhara bandha, kechari mudra, kumbhaka, and mula bandha.

- Kriya yoga: Kriya yoga involves self-study, self-discipline, and devotions.

- Sahaja yoga: Sahaja yoga teaches Kundalini activation methods to enable a person to achieve self-realization.

Yoga is considered as a structured path. These Kundalini-based Yoga forms have specific techniques for activating, maintaining, and making use of Kundalini for different purposes. You can learn Yoga on your own but to be sure you carry out the techniques properly, it's best to attend a class.

Yoga improves the interconnections between the mind and body, making you more capable of directing subtle energies at will. It will make you aware of your limitations so you can surpass them. Although the postures and movements may be difficult, they will make you familiar with how your physical, mental, and energy bodies work, and eventually, you will learn how to control them so they serve you better.

Kriya Yoga

Kriya Yoga is one form of yoga that is said to be a safer alternative to forcing the Kundalini upwards. According to Paramhansa Yogananda – a yoga master from India that brought Kundalini knowledge to the West – Kriya Yoga is a technique that combines the right attitude and purity of heart with life force stimulation so that problems are avoided.

Kriyas are "activities" and can be linked to the spontaneous movements that tend to occur upon the awakening of the Shakti. The kriyas help remove the blocks that stand in the way of the kundalini as it traverses the central channel and spine. They are triggered by the energy's interaction with the blockages.

There is a belief that the higher chakras are positive magnets that pull the consciousness upwards towards the divine, while the chakra at the spine's base pulls it downwards towards ignorance, selfishness, and materialism. In this belief system, the Kundalini is the thrust of consciousness that is related to matter, and it causes the restlessness of the mind during meditation.

The goal of guiding the Kundalini upwards is to pull it away from its negative position and unite it with the positive magnet at the top of the head. The problem is, many practices just aim to shake this energy loose. However, this energy is quite dangerous, and overstimulating it causes extreme heat that may damage the person's nervous system and cause psychological disturbances.

Kriya Yoga is safer and easier than other practices, and it can also pave the way towards spiritual enlightenment. Because it's a holistic discipline, it can improve your physical and psychological well-being. Basically, it involves the cleansing of the energy channels so that energies can move more freely in the body.

These are some of the things under Kriya Yoga that can help with awakening the energy:

- Have love for the divine. This means going beyond simply practicing religious rituals just because you are taught to do them, but having a genuine desire to commune and unite with your God.

- See everything and everyone as manifestations of the Divine. The truth is, the Universe is a part of the one who created it, so you must have respect for creation as well.

- Have a positive attitude. Although life will inevitably make you feel negative at times, do your best not to get stuck in negativity. Activating Kundalini means you have to keep your energy channels clear and your frequency high.

- Do things that cause spiritual expansion. Activities that cause upliftment to yourself and others have benefits to your spiritual condition. This could be anything such as learning a productive skill, being generous to others, helping out with a cause, etc.

- Acknowledge your higher nature. All people have lower and higher natures but not all of them live as spiritual beings. The more that you are conscious of your spiritual aspect, the better your chances are of progressing spiritually.

- Develop greater awareness. Prevent yourself from going deeper into unconsciousness by indulging in things that dull your mind. Be more mindful. Participate in meaningful and productive endeavors. Try not to do things that you know are nonsensical or detrimental to you or others.

- Chanting with a devotional attitude may raise your Kundalini. Take note that inciting mantras half-heartedly may be useless.

- Be energetic. Find things to do that give you energy. Dedicate yourself to things you are passionate about. These have effects to your subtle energies as well.

- Interestingly, waking the stored Kundalini energy can be done not only by stirring it and forcing it to shoot up from below, but it can also be coaxed upward by drawing it from above. To do this, you must make your higher chakras magnetic.

- Meditating upon saints, mystics, deities, and other spiritual personas will help you with this. By calling upon them, they may help you awaken your spirituality.

Basically, the things mentioned above can help you be in touch with your spiritual nature whether you practice Kriya yoga or not. If you want to follow the path of Kriya yoga, here's a simplified version of how to do it:

Procedure

Develop and keep a good posture. Be mindful that your spine is straight for as often as you can. This will be beneficial not only to your physical health and energy level, it may also assist your Kundalini in its ascent.

Be physically active. Kriya Yoga is all about balance, so you have to balance meditation with physical exercise. Moving your body will help with removing unclean and used energy. Aerobic exercises will invigorate you and directly help with moving the Kundalini, but you may also do mild exercises such as simple stretches, head rolls, and the like.

Sit on a chair with your feet flat, or on the floor in the crossed leg or lotus position. Keep your spine straight and your head parallel to the ground. Close your eyes and remove all distractions and preoccupations from your mind.

Focus entirely on your breath. The breath is prana, so you must be sensitive to your respirations in order to work with subtle energy. Using your mind, you will direct it to bring up the Kundalini upwards through the seven chakras that line your spine.

Feel your breath stirring in the base of your spine. You may feel it becoming warmer when you do so. This is the energy becoming activated. Just accept it and bring it upwards with each breath. Be sensitive to it. Notice what it's doing. Do not force it to move but gently coax it. It will untangle coils and burn impediments on its own.

Continue bringing your breath up until you feel energy running along your spine. When you feel that the energy has reached the topmost chakra, bring your breath down one chakra at a time until you reach the heart.

Inhale from the bottom of your spine again to bring up the energy to the crown. As you exhale, bring the energy down and let it go out of your heart. This is a more balanced form of awakening; try this if you're overwhelmed by raising Kundalini from the bottom up.

Purification

Hindu tradition requires the cleansing and strengthening of the body to prepare it for the passage of Kundalini. Fasting is sometimes prescribed - this may mean not eating for a certain number of days or not eating particular kinds of food like red meat. Activities that entertain the senses are likewise prohibited to refresh the mind and make it concentrate on spirituality.

Traditionally, kundalini awakening is done in a learning setting. There are still gurus who go handpick worthy students to impart teachings that they don't share to anybody else. Nowadays, anyone who wants

to learn may go to a guru or join a workshop.
Kundalini Spiritual Awakening

Kundalini awakenings happen differently for everyone. For some, they are slow and come in persistently but over time. For others, it can be extremely quick, almost like an explosion of energy in the gut area. Either way, Kundalini awakenings can be quite intense for anyone who experiences them.

Here are some of the symptoms you can expect to experience during your awakening.

Remember, not everyone will experience all of the same symptoms. Furthermore, you may experience some that have not been listed here. That is okay, too. The goal is to be one with the process and welcome anything that comes your way.

Everything Seems to Fall Apart

One of the first things many people experience in the face of their awakening is feelings of nervousness. As you awaken, it may feel like everything is falling apart. This is because the world as you have come to know it is being perceived through the eyes of someone who has Kundalini that is still dormant. As a result, you may feel like everything as you know it falls away.

Many people who awaken will experience massive life changes as a result of this falling apart. Several of the aspects of their lives that are not aligned with their awakened energies will begin to drift away as they make room for new, aligned experiences in their lives. Although in the long run, this is generally all for the best, in the midst of everything falling apart you can feel intense bouts of chaos and stress. Sometimes, people will even block their awakening to lessen the chaos and prevent the stress from increasing.

Everything that has been used as a crutch to support your unhealed self will begin to render themselves as useless as you realize that they are no longer supporting you. This can, of course, be scary. Many call this "leaving their comfort zone" because they are venturing beyond the system they have carefully built around themselves to bring some peace and comfort into their lives. However, they will virtually always end up finding a more pure and true sense of comfort later in their lives when they enter a later phase of their awakening.

Physical Symptoms

Many individuals that undergo awakening experience physical symptoms as a part of the process. These symptoms are generally very random and are not linked to any health issues carried by the individual. Of course, if you do experience any ongoing physical symptoms that are particularly alarming, you should always contact your physician to rule out anything serious. However, realize that if nothing comes back and you remain "undiagnosed," it is likely that these are symptoms of your awakening.

Some of the physical symptoms people experience include anything from shaking to visual disturbances. Some will also struggle to relax as a result of the major rushes of energy that course through their bodies. Others still may even experience near-death experiences that either contributes to the awakening or are a result of the awakening. Remember, whatever symptoms you experience, if you are at all concerned you should certainly contact a physician. Even though they may be spiritual awakening symptoms, it is always important to take proper precautionary methods and look after your physical body.

The reason why many people will experience physical symptoms is that their physical body is simply unable to handle such a rush of energy. As the awakening continues, these symptoms should subside. The body will grow more accustomed to the incoming energies and will likely find it significantly easier to handle. Feeling physical symptoms may encourage you to deny your awakening, but as long as you are truly healthy, enduring them can lead to powerful results. If you are particularly concerned, you can always work alongside a Kundalini master to receive support and guidance in how to manage these symptoms and potentially slow them down to make them more manageable as you endure your awakening. In general, your physical, emotional, and energetic symptoms should last only about 20 minutes at a time.

Emotional Symptoms

Emotional symptoms are extremely common in Kundalini awakenings. In fact, they are felt by virtually everyone who experiences their awakening. Emotional symptoms vary, but early on the most common symptoms include ones like anxiety, despair, and depression. The emotions can also range in the opposite direction, bringing intense feelings of elation, joy, and an overwhelming sense of peace to the individual.

These emotional fluctuations are directly the result of the changing energy within your body. At first, they may be intense and overwhelming. You may feel as though you are encountering and enduring many mood swings, which could make it challenging to deal with. The best thing that you can do is allow yourself to embody the emotions and feel through them. Refrain from blocking them or resisting them, as this can result in you directly resisting your awakening.

Energetic Symptoms

The primary energetic symptoms experiences by individuals experiencing a Kundalini awakening are massive influxes of energies at seemingly random times. These energies can become quite powerful, resulting in people randomly feeling extremely energized and even restless. These energy symptoms are inevitable, as spiritual awakenings do exist in the non-physical life-force energy of Kundalini. You may experience many symptoms as a result. Virtually all emotional and physical symptoms stem from the energetic symptoms of your awakening.

One interesting aspect of energetic symptoms is that many will go unnoticed. Because these are less tangible than physical and emotional symptoms, many things will actually go on in the background that will contribute to your overall shift. The best thing you can do to manage energetic symptoms is to find peace, allow them to flow, and work through anything that they bring your way either physically or energetically. The more you allow them to move through, the better it will become for you.

Importance of breathing in meditation and yoga

Take a full breath, growing your midsection. Delay. Breathe out gradually to the count of five. Do this multiple times.

Congrats. You've recently calmed your nervous system.

Controlled breathing, similar to what you basically practiced, has been seen to lessen stress, increase readiness and lift your spirits. For quite a long time, yogis have used breath control, or pranayama, to increase focus and improve imperativeness. Buddha supported breath-meditation as an approach to arrive at enlightenment.

Science is merely starting to give proof that the advantages of this ancient practice are genuine. Studies have found, for instance, that breathing practices can help lessen side effects related to tension, a sleeping disorder, post-traumatic stress issues, depression and a lack of ability to concentrate consistently scatter.

Intelligent Breathing

If you have the opportunity to learn just a single system, this is the one to try. In sound breathing, the objective is to inhale at a pace of five breaths for each minute, which by and large converts into breathing in and breathing out to the count of six. If you have never worked on breathing activities, you may need to work up to this training gradually, beginning with breathing in and breathing out to the count of three and making your way up to six.

1. Sitting up straight or resting, place your hands on your tummy.

2. Gradually breathe in, extending your tummy, to the count of five.

3. Rest.

4. Gradually inhale out to the count of six.

5. Make your way up to doing this 10 to 20 minutes every day.

Stress Relief

At the point when your brain is busy, or you are stressed, try Rock and Roll breathing, which has the additional advantage of reinforcing your centre.

1. Sit up straight on the floor or on the edge of a seat.

2. Place your hands on your gut.

3. As you breathe in, lean forward and extend your gut.

4. As you breathe out, press the breath out and twist forward while inclining in reverse; breathe out until you're empty of breath.

5. Repeat several times.

Empowering HA Breath

When the midafternoon droop hits, stand up and do some quick breathwork to awaken your soul and body.

1. Stand up tall, elbows bowed, palms pointing up.

2. As you breathe in, move your elbows back behind you, palms still pointed up.

3. At that point breathe out rapidly, pushing your palms forward and turning them downward,

while at the same time saying "Ha" so anyone can hear.

4. Repeat rapidly 10 or more times.

Chapter 3: The Energy of Prana

Prana is a Sanskrit word that deciphers as "imperative life power." Understanding what prana is and how it functions resembles being given a key that can open new improved degrees of wellbeing and prosperity—on the all around.

Prana is the widespread ocean of vitality that imbues and vitalizes all issue. This ocean of vitality combines into sub-nuclear particles and molecules, which become the essential structure squares of all issue showing the physical world. Along these lines, each particle, atom, and cell is an expansion of prana, similarly as waves are augmentations of the ocean that lies underneath them.

The five fundamental resources of our tendency—the brain, breath (prana), discourse, hearing, and sight—were contending about which was the most significant. To determine the question they chose that each would leave the body thus to see whose nonappearance was missed most. First discourse left, yet the body kept on thriving however it was quiet. Next the eye left, yet the body thrived however visually impaired. At that point the ear left, yet the body flourished however hard of hearing. At last the mind left, yet still the body lived on, however it was presently oblivious. Be that as it may, the minute the prana began to leave, the body started to bite the dust. Different resources were quickly losing their life-power, so they all raced to prana, conceded its amazingness, and implored it to remain.

This is an old Vedic story, marginally various renditions of which are found in different Upanishads. The contention in the first place speaks to the common human condition where our resources are not incorporated, however rival each other for control of our consideration. When prana leaves, it turns out to be certain that prana offers vitality to every one of our resources, without which none of them can work. Along these lines the lesson of this story is that to control these resources, one must control the prana.

To achieve positive changes in body and mind we should comprehend the vitality through which they work. This power is called prana in Sanskrit, signifying "essential vitality," once in a while deciphered as "breath" or "fundamental power," however it is really something more. The various structures through which prana communicates are only from time to time inspected inside and out in Western writing on yoga, and therefore the study of prana, which is tremendous and significant, is once in a while comprehended.

Prana has numerous degrees of significance, from the physical breath to the vitality of awareness itself. Prana isn't just the essential life-constrain, it is the first inventive power. It is the ace type of all vitality working at each degree of our being. Without a doubt the whole universe is a sign of prana. Indeed, even kundalini shakti, the snake control or inward vitality which changes our cognizance, creates from stirred prana.

On a vast level there are two parts of prana. The first is unmanifest, the vitality of unadulterated cognizance, which rises above all creation. The second, or show prana, is simply the power of creation.

Nature itself is made out of three gunas, or characteristics: sattva, or agreement, which offers ascend to the brain; rajas, or development, which offers ascend to prana; and tamas, or idleness, which offers ascend to the physical body. Nature is a functioning, or rajasic, vitality. Reacting to the draw of the higher Self, or unadulterated cognizance, this vitality progresses toward becoming sattvic. By the inactivity of numbness this equivalent vitality progresses toward becoming tamasic.

Comparative with our physical presence, prana or crucial vitality is an alteration of the air component, getting principally from the oxygen we relax. On an unobtrusive level, the air component relates to the feeling of touch; through touch we feel invigorated and can transmit our life-power to other people.

Prana is additionally the power that streams in every living structure and performs crucial capacities. Paramhansa Yogananda called this part of prana "life-power." He further clarified that life-power has a characteristic insight empowering it to do the life-continuing procedures.

To offer lucidity to this picture, he even begat the expression "lifetrons." We have an inconspicuous or astral body made up of prana that underlies the physical body. Oriental recuperating methods, for example, Ayurveda and needle therapy, work to fit and fortify the progression of life-power, calling it differently prana, chi, or ki. At the point when the life-power streams appropriately, the outcome will be a characteristic condition of wellbeing and imperativeness.

Prana is additionally used to allude to the breath. At the point when we take a physical breath, there is a relating development of prana in the unpretentious or astral spine. Prana streams up in the inconspicuous spine related to the inward breath, and down with the exhalation.

This connection among breath and the progression of prana is integral to a significant number of the strategies of contemplation. By controlling the breath, which is effectively felt, we can impact the progression of prana, which is considerably more inconspicuous and hard to feel.

The Koshas

The person comprises of five koshas or "sheaths":

1.Annamaya kosha ("sheath made of nourishment"). This is the physical body, made out of the five components we ingest (earth, water, air, fire, ether).

2.Pranamaya kosha ("sheath made of breath"). This is the fundamental body, made out of five parts of prana called vayus.

3.Manomaya kosha ("sheath of impressions"). This is the external, or lower level, of psyche, loaded up with the five sorts of tactile impressions.

4.Vijnanamaya kosha ("sheath of thoughts"). This is knowledge itself, coordinated mental action.

5.Anandamaya kosha ("sheath of encounters"). This is the more profound personality, containing the memory, subliminal personality, and superconscious mind.

The pranamaya kosha is an amazing circle energies. This sheath intercedes between the physical body on one side and the three sheaths of the psyche (external personality, knowledge, and internal personality) on the other. It likewise intercedes between the five gross components and the five tangible impressions.

Pranayama (prana = vitality + yama = control) is a kind of contemplation method that includes different methods for controlling the breathing, with the objective being to raise one's prana (additionally called Kundalini for this situation) up the profound spine to the otherworldly eye or 6th chakra, which carries one to illumination. Kriya Yoga is one such procedure, made surely understood by Paramhamsa Yogananda in Autobiography of a Yogi.

How Pranayama Works

On either side of the spine there is a fiery nerve channel, or nadi : ida on the left and pingala on the right.

The prana or vitality ventures upward through the ida nadi. With this upward development, the breath is consequently drawn into the lungs. Accordingly, the psyche is attracted outward to the universe of the faculties.

The vitality at that point voyages downwards through the pingala nadi. At the point when the vitality is going down, it is called apana instead of prana. This descending development is joined by physical exhalation, and connotes a dismissal of outer conditions.

One indication of this cycle is the relationship of inward breath with fervor and bliss, and exhalation with annihilation and despondency. Joy and misery should consistently pursue each other when the reason for each is outer conditions, which are continually evolving.

Be that as it may, through pranayama procedures an individual can rather divert the vitality through the profound spine in the middle of the ida and pingala, called the sushumna. At the point when the degree of vitality in the sushumna arrives at the highest point of the spine and goes into the profound eye, or 6th chakra, one ends up illuminated.

The vast majority of us are commanded by the fundamental body and its profound situated urges, which are essential with the goal for us to stay alive. The essential body is the home of the subliminal self image, which harbors our different feelings of trepidation, wants, and connections. A large portion of us consume our time on earth looking for happiness through this kosha as tactile delight and procuring material articles.

Individuals with a solid imperative body can intrigue their character on the world and frequently become conspicuous throughout everyday life. Those with a feeble fundamental body don't have the vitality to achieve a lot, and typically stay in subordinate positions. For the most part individuals with solid yet self absorbed essential natures run the world. However, this nature can be perhaps the best impediment on the profound way since it makes it hard for the individual to give up to any higher power or to scrutinize their own craving based driving forces.

This makes a few people think profound life expects us to stifle our prana, yet a solid pranamaya kosha is very unique in relation to prideful or want arranged essentialness. It gets its quality not from individual power however from our give up to the vitality of the awesome. Without a solid spiritualized pranamaya kosha, we come up short on the vitality to do our practices in an extraordinary and continued way.

In Hindu folklore this higher prana is symbolized by the monkey god Hanuman, child of the breeze, whose story is told in the antiquated Indian exemplary the Ramayana. Hanuman gave up to the heavenly as the celestial manifestations Rama and his better half, Sita, and he along these lines picked up the capacity to progress toward becoming as huge or as little as he wished, to conquer all adversaries and deterrents, and to achieve the wonderful. Such a profoundly coordinated crucial nature has vitality, interest, and eagerness, alongside the capacity to control the faculties and indispensable urges—all subordinate to a higher will and goal.

The Five Pranas in Yoga

The pranamaya kosha is made out of the five pranas, likewise called vayus or "powers of the air." These five pranas are sorted by development and bearing. This is a significant point in Ayurvedic drug just as in yogic practices.

Prana Vayu

•Prana vayu actually signifies "forward-moving air," since it moves internal and administers a wide range of gathering into the body, from eating, drinking, and breathing in, to the gathering of tangible impressions and mental encounters. It is propulsive in nature, getting things under way and directing them, and it gives the fundamental vitality that drives us throughout everyday life.

Apana Vayu

•Apana vayu, "the air that moves away," moves descending and outward, overseeing all types of end and propagation (which additionally has a descending development). It administers the end of stool and pee, the ousting of semen, menstrual liquid, and the embryo, and the end of carbon dioxide through the breath. On a more profound level, it controls the end of negative tactile, passionate, and mental encounters. It is the premise of our insusceptible capacity.

Udana Vayu

•Udana vayu, "the upward-moving air," goes up and achieves subjective or transformative developments of the life-vitality. It administers the development of the body and the capacity to remain, just as discourse, exertion, excitement, and will. It is our principle positive vitality, helping us to build up our various sheaths and to develop in cognizance.

Samana Vayu

•Samana vayu, "adjusting air," moves from the fringe to the middle, through a beating and perceiving activity. It helps absorption on all levels, working in the gastrointestinal tract to process nourishment, in the lungs to process air or assimilate oxygen, and in the brain to process understanding—tactile, passionate, and mental.

Vyana Vayu

•Vyana vayu, "outward-moving air," moves from the middle to the fringe, overseeing dissemination on all levels. It moves nourishment, water, and oxygen all through the body, and keeps our feelings and contemplations circling in the brain, conferring energy and giving quality.

The five pranas can likewise be found as far as their body area. Prana vayu oversees the development of vitality starting from the head to the navel, which is the pranic focus of the physical body. Apana vayu oversees the development of vitality starting from the navel to the root chakra at the base of the spine. Samana vayu oversees the development of vitality from the whole body back to the navel. Vyana vayu administers the development of vitality out from the navel all through the whole body. Udana vayu oversees the development of vitality from the navel up to the head

In a nutshell, prana vayu administers the admission of substances, samana oversees their processing, and vyana oversees the dissemination of supplements. Udana administers the arrival of positive vitality, and apana oversees the end of waste materials. This is a lot of like the working of a proficient machine. Prana acquires the fuel, samana changes over this fuel to vitality, and vyana courses the vitality to different worksites. Apana discards the waste items delivered by the transformation procedure. Udana deals with the vitality along these lines made, empowering the machine to work viably.

The way to wellbeing is to keep our pranas working in congruity. At the point when one prana winds up imbalanced, the others will in general lose their balance too, in light of the fact that they are altogether connected. For the most part prana and udana balance apana, as the powers of empowerment balance those of disposal. Essentially vyana and samana organize with one another regarding development and constriction.

How Prana Creates the Physical Body

Without prana the physical body is close to a piece of earth. Prana shapes this thick mass into different appendages and organs by making different unpretentious nerve channels, or nadis, through which it can work and stimulate gross issue, molding it into different tissues and organs.

Prana vayu makes the openings and diverts in the head and mind down to the heart. There are seven openings in the head: the two eyes, two ears, two nostrils, and mouth. Udana vayu helps prana in making the openings in the upper piece of the body, especially the mouth and vocal organs, in light of the fact that the mouth is the principle opening for the head as well as for the whole body. Indeed, the physical body is, one might say, an expansion of the mouth, which is simply the primary organ of eating and articulation.

Prana and the Mind

Mental vitality is gotten from nourishment, breath, and the impressions we take in from the outside world. Prana administers the admission of tactile impressions, samana oversees their psychological processing, and vyana administers mental dissemination. Apana rules the disposal of poisonous thoughts and negative feelings. Udana gives positive mental vitality, quality, and excitement.

On a mental level, prana oversees our receptivity to positive wellsprings of sustenance, feeling, and learning through the brain and faculties. At the point when unsettled it causes unfortunate wants and unquenchable yearnings, and we become confused, misled, and by and large out of equalization.

Apana oversees our capacity to dispense with negative contemplations and feelings. At the point when unhinged it causes despondency, and we get stopped up with undigested experience that overloads us throughout everyday life, making us dreadful, smothered, and powerless.

Samana gives us sustenance, satisfaction, and a fair personality. At the point when disturbed it realizes connection and covetousness. We stick to things and become contracted, stale, and possessive in our conduct.

Vyana gives free development and autonomy of psyche. At the point when unsettled it can cause detachment, disdain, and distance. We become incapable to join with others or to stay associated with what we are doing.

Udana gives us bliss and eagerness and stirs our higher profound and innovative possibilities. At the point when disturbed it can cause pride and self-importance, and we become ungrounded, attempting to go excessively high and putting some distance between our foundations.

Profound Aspects of the Pranas

The pranas have numerous uncommon capacities in yogic practices. On an otherworldly level, samana oversees the space inside the heart wherein the genuine Self abides as a fire with seven blazes. Samana manages our internal fire, which must consume equitably. Without the harmony and equalization samana makes, we can't come back profoundly of our being or concentrate our brain.

Vyana oversees the development of prana through the nadis, keeping them open, clear, clean, and even in their working. Apana shields us from negative astral impacts and fanciful encounters. Prana vayu gives us the best possible desire essential for profound improvement.
Udana oversees our development in cognizance and conveys the psyche into the conditions of imagining and profound rest, and into the after-death domains. Udana additionally oversees development up the sushumna. Since the mind moves with udana vayu, it is commonly the most significant prana for profound development.

As we practice yoga, the unobtrusive parts of these pranas start to stir, which may cause different unordinary developments of vitality in body and brain, including different unconstrained developments called kriyas. We may feel new scopes of vitality (unpretentious vyana); extraordinary harmony (unobtrusive samana); a feeling of delicacy, as though we are suspending (inconspicuous udana); profound groundedness and steadiness (unobtrusive apana); or just increased imperativeness and affectability (unobtrusive prana).

Working with Prana

Legitimate sustenance increments prana on a physical level. Appropriate end likewise makes a difference. In Ayurvedic thought, the prana from nourishment is invested in the internal organ, especially in the upper 66% of this organ. Hence apana is the most significant prana for physical wellbeing.

The Vedas state that humans eat nourishment with apana, while the divine beings eat nourishment with prana. The humans are the physical tissues, continued by right nourishment. The immortals are the faculties that take in nourishment by means of prana itself as tactile impressions. To reinforce prana, practices, for example, customs and perceptions are significant, just as tangible treatments including shading, sounds, or fragrances, and contact with nature.

The principle approach to work with prana is through pranayama, especially as yogic breathing activities. Yoga underlines refinement of both body and psyche as a way to Self-acknowledgment, and therefore it accentuates a veggie lover diet rich in prana—that is, nourishments brimming with the life-power—and a brain established in moral qualities, for example, honesty and peacefulness, and in otherworldly teaches. An unclean, lethal, or upset body and psyche can't understand the higher Self. The way to cleaning body and brain is prana, which connections the two. The principle strategy is refinement of the nadis through which prana streams.

While all yogic breathing activities are useful in such manner, the most significant is nadi shodhana (interchange nostril breathing), which enables parity to right and left prana flows. As per the yogic framework, the body and every one of its channels have a privilege or left transcendence. The correct side is sun based in nature. It helps in such exercises as processing, work, and focus, and is pittic, or searing, in constitution. The left, or the lunar, nadi is kaphic, or water prevalent. It helps in such exercises as rest, rest, and unwinding.

Ordinary exchange nostril breathing is the most significant strategy for keeping our pranas or energies in equalization, yet there is another technique— joining prana and apana. Apana vayu, which is lined up with the power of gravity, as a rule moves descending, coming about in malady and passing as well as in the descending development of awareness. Prana vayu, then again, will in general scatter upward through the brain and faculties, and is our pathway to the energies above. Yogic practices require bringing apana up and cutting prana down so the two can join together; this helps balance all the pranas. In doing as such, the inward fire or kundalini winds up enkindled in the area of the navel. Mula bandha (the root lock) is a significant practice in such manner.

Mantra and Meditation

The pranas in the psyche can be managed legitimately. There are pranayama systems that work with the psyche and faculties, and are not simply constrained to the breath. Shading and sound (music) are significant approaches to coordinate vitality in the psyche, however the best method is mantra, especially single syllable, or bija, mantras like Om, which make vibrations that can help direct positive vitality into the subliminal. Reflection itself, making space in the psyche, serves to make more prana, and when the brain is brought into a quiet and open condition, similar to a region of sky, another vitality appears which can realize incredible change.

Every one of the ways of yoga depend on controlling prana. Bhakti yoga, or the yoga of dedication, achieves pranic change by joining us with the perfect prana. Karma yoga, or administration, depends on arrangement with the awesome will, which likewise gives us more prana, not exclusively to act apparently, however for internal improvement.

Old style yoga, or raja yoga, depends on the control of mental exercises (chitta vrittis). The vibration of the psyche (chitta spanda) pursues the vibration of (prana spanda), and in this manner pranayama helps control the brain. It additionally helps control the faculties (pratyahara), in light of the fact that it pulls back our mindfulness internal from the faculties. Hatha yoga itself is chiefly worried about prana; yoga stances happen as an outflow of pranic development, and numerous incredible yogis learned yoga stances not through mechanical practice, yet through the intensity of their stirred prana.

Jnana yoga, or the yoga of learning, requires a solid will and focus. In this yoga the prana of request must be made, which means we should ask into our actual nature, not only rationally however in the majority of our day by day exercises; without well-created udana vayu we will fail.

Undoubtedly, as the Vedas state, we are altogether under the influence of prana. Prana is the sun that gives life and light to everybody and abides inside the heart as the Self all things considered. The prana in us gives us life and enables us to act. We should figure out how to be available to and welcome this more noteworthy power and look to bring it all the more completely into our life and activities. This is perhaps the best mystery of yoga.

Getting Energy and the Pranic Body

In our physical body, blood moves through veins, vessels, and corridors. In our vitality body, prana courses through vitality pathways called nadis (nadi interprets as stream).

Prana rides on the breath, so when we take in, we take in prana. At the point when we extend the breath and improve its nature, we are growing and improving the nature of this fundamental life power inside and around us. This is actually what yoga breathing strategies, or pranayama, are intended to do.

A significant part of the pranic body are the chakras, or vitality focuses. In yoga, we center around the seven significant chakras that exist along the line of the spine, every one associated with explicit organs and organs of the physical body, just as territories of our mind that impact our character.

It is accepted by numerous that wellbeing and prosperity comes when there is a fair vitality move through every one of the seven significant chakras.

On the flipside, when prana is kept from streaming normally, either getting to be blocked or overactive at one point, it can make disharmony on both a physical and passionate level.
How Might We Help Prana Flow Freely?

By rehearsing Yoga, obviously!

Yoga stances, especially the conventional or old style asanas, initiate explicit chakras. For instance, Bridge Pose and Shoulder Stand work the vitality at the throat chakra, which can impact how we speak with others.

On a physical level, the throat chakra relates to the thyroid and parathyroid organs, and can along these lines have a supporting and adjusting impact on our digestion.

How about we not overlook pranayama, the yoga breathing procedures which are explicitly intended to grow prana. The word yama intends to control, so when we grow and control the breath, we can deliberately extend and convey the essential life power inside our framework.

While you don't really need to completely grasp this part of yoga to get the advantages, rehearsing with vigorous affectability can add another measurement to your training, and maybe help you appreciate increasingly adjusted degrees of wellbeing and prosperity.

How to comprehend prana?

1. Increase prana. You need more prana no matter what.

2. Conserve prana. You need to profit and set aside cash.

3. Channel prana. You need to spend it admirably. Use it, yet channel it.

4. Balance prana. A great deal of issue originates from awkwardness. Vitality is wild a lot of this, an excessive amount of that.

5. Purify prana. It resembles you change your 5 dollar notes to 100 dollar notes. You need to cause the

vitality to turn out to be all the more dominant. Since when it turns out to be increasingly unadulterated it turns out to be all the more dominant.

Comprehend why we are worn out

•Sometimes we think "I'm worn out so I rest". Be that as it may, reflection around then is better.

•You do the asanas so you can sit to reflect. In the end on the off chance that you will have the option to control the brain, you tune to the supernatural self.

•When you are drained, you think just about the physical body, however you are not understanding that your tiredness is additionally originating from mental tiredness and profound tiredness.

•When you are drained you think just about the physical body and state " I would be advised to go get some nourishment". That implies you allude back over and over to the physical body.

•But you additionally have mental tiredness, mental enthusiastic tiredness. At the point when you are drained perhaps you have the psychological tiredness since you have some negative feelings that are gobbling you up inside.

•You probably won't know about that. Like you resent something or you detest something and your astuteness go off course thinking all sort of things that are totally off-base.

•On top of that, the personality is there, obstructing the stream, so the vitality of unadulterated cognizance isn't there, and you are blocking yourself from that progression of vitality.

The Prana Pulse

•We need to figure out how to feel the beat of our prana consistently and when we feel that our prana is deficient with regards to, you have the decision to go to the most elevated wellspring of prana, the profound prana . This most perfect sort of prana that will supply prana to the various levels.

•Any measure of physical movement won't supply the otherworldly prana and unwinding that you need. Be that as it may, on the off chance that you can yield the profound prana, this will give all of you the vitality to illuminate all your psychological, enthusiastic blockages, all your numbness in your reasoning, break up the self image and give wellbeing to the body.

•But in the event that you tune just to the physical level and decipher everything physically, focusing as long as you can remember and awareness around the physical body, you are incorrect. Around then you starve your psychological body and otherworldly body. You don't think about otherworldly reason. You put the profound behind the physical.

•So that is not an exceptionally savvy method for utilizing the Universal vitality accessible to you for your prosperity. Keep in mind, our prosperity is physical, mental, and enthusiastic.
Expanding prana

•You increment prana by a cautious decision of way of life. Way of life should be adjusted and healthy. Know about the way that the vitality of Nature originates from the vitality of the 5 fundamental components of Nature: Earth, water, fire, air, and ether.

•Just the way that you are living in nature, you are getting prana. On the off chance that you live falsely, you are cutting off yourself from the regular progression of prana. You live in solid, glass, and steel, neon light, no prana air. You go to mall, place of business, blend with numerous individuals of no insight, without supernatural considerations. Everybody is focused, and avaricious. You attempt to make cash to be someone. You leave structures and step in the vehicle and drive on expressway, the greater part of your day by day exercises are counterfeit. This way of life increments vata, and the counterfeit ness in the brain. You land at counterfeit home, eat fake nourishment, microwave. You surf the Internet and have fake connections. Would you be able to envision... ..

•You need to sustain the physical body with nature, sit on earth, see trees, embrace a tree, take a gander at creatures. Wonder about bloom, grass. This gives you prana. Attempt to monitor, don't spend. You have to settle on a shrewd decision of way of life which will give you energy and aliveness. Some of the time, you have to settle on extraordinary decisions to recover your personal satisfaction.

Saving prana

•When you are debilitated, you lie there and you can't talk, think, or move, in light of the fact that your prana is totally down. Envision everything takes prana. Throughout the day you are dynamic you are moving near. You are thinking. You go through so much prana. How would you energize? You can't spend more than you make.

•Daily, you need to compute in your mind brisk how would you spend vitality. Am I accomplishing things today to energize? Consistently, you address with difficulties and you have to ration vitality spent on pointless things so you will have vitality to address with your difficulties.

•When you invest time at the ashram, you are in certainty contributing your vitality to get the profound vitality, the intelligence. On the off chance that you get this otherworldly vitality, you will squander less your vitality.

•For model, on the off chance that you have a psychological issue, when you have profound vitality, you will say "this is peanuts, this is simple" . By and large, you need point of view of your life and what your identity is. If not, you get furious of each seemingly insignificant detail. We spend vitality going round, round, round.

•Sometimes you are worn out, you would state " I'm going to eat,and visit and not go to satsang" . This implies you are not contributing carefully your vitality. Be careful not to squander your vitality on things that are redundant.

•That's the reason in yoga theory the shrewd instructor says: segregate, separate! … Don't stress, don't stress. So you can get to the wellspring of the issue. A similar issue will be there, yet you can perceive the truth about it.

Directing prana

•Channeling vitality means make your life helpful. Utilize your vitality for benevolent reason, at that point you will acquire profound vitality. On the off chance that you spend vitality for egotistical reason, it makes you feel solid, yet you pay in another way, stress, protectiveness, accumulating, prideful desire. It squares you so you pay the cost. It' s not in any case justified, despite all the trouble on the off chance that you consider appropriately.

•If you use vitality sacrificially, suppose in administration, you get the profound vitality. You utilize your physical, mental vitality, yet you receive consequently profound vitality. That is known as the guideline of karma yoga. It's a cognizant trade of vitality. It winds up profound vitality.

Adjusting prana

•How you can be imbalanced? Lets state you do an excessive amount of physical work, you won't have enough vitality for deduction and won't have the option to do mental work or even have feeling.

•Some other individuals are feeling constantly, they are enthusiastic to the point that they have no vitality for speculation. They simply feel, feel, and feel. Other individuals are thinking, thinking, and after that they have no vitality for feelings. So you should adjust everything.

•It is said on the off chance that you are excessively enthusiastic, you would need to be increasingly normal, and think a tad. In the opposite, on the off chance that an individual is excessively dry, at that point they have to build up their ability of inclination. So whatever you do at the ashram you are adjusting yourself. Serenade a bit, think a bit, tune to the profound, and monitor your physical vitality. In the event that you don't want to recite, that is actually when you have to recite to renew your enthusiastic vitality that is down and dry around then.

•This will develop that reverential vitality that floods you and adjust you and make you feel invigorated. At that point at times you would prefer not to think. Around then you should be alert and think. So you practice your scholarly vitality.

•Sometimes you need to peruse 5 hours per day. In the ashram you need to do physical work, on the grounds that a large portion of us are excessively mental. You need to go hack wood, convey water, burrow channel, clean lake. This kind of physical work is likewise useful for individuals with a lot of physical vitality as it would spend that abundance of physical vitality out and balance you. Else you become out of sort.

A few people are so assimilated at taking a gander at their neighbor for example they are self-retained, constantly stressed over others' opinion of them. This proud vitality devours them. We have to have enough of mindfulness, yet in the event that you are devoured by it, around then you become cut off from your higher reason.

Cleanse prana

•This is the most intriguing theme. How would you purge your vitality? You decontaminate through rehearsing otherworldly practices, by deliberately going in a direction of how to manage your body, mind, feelings that is helping you to change cognizance. That is called sadhana. That is the manner by which you sanitize your vitality.

•Practicing sadhana isn't your typical inclination. In any case, when you comprehend the pattern of your body – mind and see how you continue rehashing examples and make botches, around then, you attempt to prepare your body-mind distinctively and move it from its typical course.

•Sadhana expels the inner self and it moves toward becoming cleaned. Sadhana changes your wavelength from gross to unpretentious. In yoga, each training is to sanitize your entire framework. Your nadis become clear, and more vitality moves through.

•Sw. Sivananda says it is imperative to sanitize our considerations. How to do this? One of the practices is satsanga, when you go to the individuals who skill to think and you hear them out then you consider what they said. The possibility of decontamination is we are unadulterated soul unadulterated Self.

•Everything about us is emanating unadulterated vitality. We have huge measure of prana or vitality and the principle is the profound vitality. We have it in bounty. Everything else we do is simply to clean the covering that is deterring that brilliance of the Self that is as of now inside us. The more you increase Self-information or Self-mindfulness the more vitality or prana you get.

Chapter 4: Psychic Abilities

Psychic abilities are said to be supernatural powers. These are abilities that others would consider impossible. However, it should be noted that psychic abilities are possible and that there are people who possess such abilities. In fact, every human being possesses some psychic abilities to a certain degree. The problem is that most people do not develop their abilities. Consequently, they are not able to use and take advantage of their abilities. If only people could take more time to meditate, then you will see that psychic abilities are supposed to be very common. In fact, regular practice of even the basic breathing meditation can help you awaken your latent psychic abilities.

From now on, you should not see psychic abilities as something that is extraordinary. Realize that you possess these abilities. It is just a matter of developing and making use of your abilities. Yes, you need to learn to use them effectively.

Psychic abilities have become controversial. In fact, there are those who completely do not believe in the existence of such abilities. This is due to the sad fact that those who surface and claim to possess psychic abilities are mere hacks and scams who do not even know how to meditate. Do not allow these people to discourage you from pursuing a noble and magical path. After all, the best way for you to ensure that such abilities truly exist is by seeing it for yourself. The more that you meditate, the more that you will realize the psychic abilities that you possess.

The different psychic abilities

There are numerous psychic abilities in the world. Although it would be great to master all of them, it would be practical to just find which ability you prefer the most and use your time and efforts to master that ability. If you can dedicate more time, then you can branch out and learn another ability. Keep in mind that when it comes to learning, you need to focus on the quality of your learning. So, feel free to learn as many psychic abilities as you want, but be sure not to sacrifice the quality of your learning.

So, what are the different psychic abilities? Well, there are many. One of the most heard of is clairvoyance. Clairvoyance or clear-seeing is the ability to see beyond what the physical eyes can see. It can allow you to look beyond and divine the future, see and read auras, as well as see subtle energies and entities, among others. The ability of clairvoyance is closely related to your ajna chakra, which is the seat of intuition and higher consciousness. If you want to develop this psychic ability, then you need to develop your ajna chakra.

Another psychic ability that you should know is known as clairsentience, which means clear feeling. It refers to the ability to receive intuitive messages through emotions and feelings, which may also include physical sensations. People who have this ability are often referred to as empaths. This is due to their ability known as empathy. This ability will allow you to feel people and understand them on a much deeper level. This is characterized by a heightened sensitivity to subtle energies, feelings, and emotions. The more that you engage in meditation, the more that you can develop this ability. To be more specific, this ability is more associated with the heart chakra. Of course, the ajna chakra also has an important role to play in the development of this psychic ability.

Clairaudience refers to clear hearing. Think of it like a little voice that tells you the right thing to do. You are probably aware of the saying that there is an angel beside you that sometimes tells you the right thing to do. Well, many times, it is actually the psychic ability known as clairaudience that should be given credit. This ability is also linked to the ajna chakra as it makes use of the intuition. It is also worth noting that messages from the spiritual world are often received through this psychic ability. You cannot expect for those in the spiritual plane to manifest strongly in the physical plane, as they are in a different realm or plane of existence.

Almost everyone has a good memory of some experience with this psychic ability. It is that "voice" that speaks in your head and tells you the right thing to do or idea to think about. You might think of it as the messages from your guardian angel. Although it is true that we can receive messages from our guardian angel, it is also true that some of these meaningful messages may come not from an angel but from your intuition and is communicated to you in a psychic way. The more that you do meditation, the more that you will be able to notice this "voice" in your head. It is your intuition talking to you. Listen to it.

Another interesting psychic ability is known as claircognizance, also known as clear knowing. It is the ability to just know things even without any logic or fact. You can consider it as some kind of inner knowing. For example, having this "knowing" that you should not trust a certain person, only to find out that that person really cannot be trusted or is a bad person. Take note that this is different from clairaudience. In this case, there is no voice of any kind that you have to deal with. Instead, you simply know things as they are. You do not have to do anything; you just know. Although all your chakras should be well developed to master this ability, there are two main chakras that are primarily needed for this psychic ability: the crown chakra and the ajna chakra.

However, it should be noted that there are many other psychic abilities that exist. Unfortunately, the world only considers the above abilities to be the "main" abilities. The truth is that there are many other abilities that are just as wonderful.

Telekinesis

Telekinesis is the psychic ability to move objects using the power of the mind. This is one of the most fascinating abilities that you can learn. It is also very popular. However, the question remains: Is it real? The answer to this is *yes*. However, learning telekinesis takes time and practice. If you want to learn telekinesis, then here are the instructions that you need:

Place a light object in front of you, preferably on a table. You can use a feather, small stone, or anything that is light enough. Now, just relax. Focus on the object in front of you. Now, visualize forming a tunnel between you and the object. Nothing should exist in front of you but the object of your focus. Now, visualize your astral hand reaching out and pushing the object. Another thing that you can do is to visualize a ray of prana pushing the object. Watch it move.

As you can see, the steps are simple. It is up to you to practice this technique until you are able to do it properly. Once you get good at it, you can skip the part where you have to envision a tunnel between you and the object. After all, its purpose is only to aid you in your visualization and give you better focus.

Here is another technique that you can use to do telekinesis:

Place an object in front of you. Just relax. Now, focus on the object. Try to feel the object. Be one with it. Consider the object to be an extension of yourself. How does it feel to be the object? Do you feel how it (you) is attached to the table? Be one with it. The more that you become one with it, the more that you can feel that you can move it, much like when you try to move your hand. When you finally reach the point where you are, indeed, one with the object – that you are the object – then just move, and it will move.

It is important to be one with the object to the point that you feel that the object has become a part of you. Another thing to take note of is not to use force. When you practice telekinesis, you need to be relaxed. A common mistake is to use force when you focus on something. Take note that focusing does not mean that you need to use force. The more relaxed you are, the better. The important thing is your state of mind.

Telekinesis is actually divided into two categories: microkinesis and microkinesis. The two techniques above are examples of macrokinesis whereby you actually move objects. If you think that it is too difficult for you, then you might want to start out with microkinesis. Microkinesis deals with randomness instead of literally moving objects with your mind.

Here is an exercise that you can do to try microkinesis.

Use a random generator. You can also use a die or a coin if you want. Microkinesis is about influencing the outcome of randomness. Instead of making an object move, you should create a certain outcome. For example, flip a coin and make it land with the head side facing up. You can also shuffle a deck of cards and use your ability to make the top card always a red card. Again, microkinesis is about influencing the result of randomness. So, how do you do this? It is similar to moving an object. For this exercise, let us use a die. The objective is to make it land on the number 6 (the number 6 facing up). The steps are as follows:

Relax and hold the die in your hand. Before you roll the die, visualize that the outcome of the will be number 6. Visualize this repeatedly in your mind. Feel the die in your hand and be one with it. You will have this feeling that you are one with the die and that you can, indeed, control it to roll to any number that you want. Now, roll the die with certainty that the outcome will be the number of your choice. In this case, it is number 6. You can also try a different number.

Feel free to device your own method or exercise. The principle remains the same: You should use visualization and be one with the object. Once again, never use any kind of force. Keep in mind that you do not force things to happen; instead, you just let things happen.

Pyrokinesis

Pyrokinesis is another psychic ability that will allow you to control fire. Indeed, many people would want to learn this technique. Just like any other kinetic ability, pyrokinesis takes effort to learn, but it is worth practicing. For this exercise, you will need to use a candle. The steps are as follows:

Light the candle. Relax. Now, focus on the flame of the candle. Be one with it. Feel it. Feel yourself as the flame. Do you feel how hot you are? This flame is an extension of yourself. Spend some more time becoming one with the flame. Once you reach this point of oneness with the flame, you can easily feel that you can move it. Make it lean to one side, and then to the other. Remember: you are the flame.

To move the candle flame, you might also want to use visualization. If you truly become one with the flame, you will notice that you do not need to exert too much effort. You can just feel it and will it to move. Once again, the same principles apply—merging with the object and visualization. If you get good at it, you might not even have to use visualization. This depends on your spiritual maturity, as well as how much your personal preference. The best way to find out what will work for you is to try it out and see for yourself.

However, doing so would require another book, or even books, to cover everything. For now, you have the information that you need that can help you activate and develop your psychic senses. Let us now move on and discuss what is known as psychic awareness.

Psychic awareness

Psychic awareness is not a psychic ability per se but more about the right approach that you need to take when you awaken your psychic senses. As the saying goes, "With great power come great responsibilities." If you are just starting out, you might consider your psychic senses to be quite strange. This is because you are not yet used to them. However, the more that you do the meditation techniques in this book, the more that you will be in touch with your psychic senses. Soon enough, they will be very common and normal for you. Since meditation empowers all the chakras, you can rest for sure that you will develop several psychic senses/abilities if you religiously practice the techniques in this book.

When it comes to being aware, it is important to be aware of the presence of energy, as well as the quality of this energy. For example, if you meet someone and sense a strong negative energy, then you might want to avoid that person, or at least put up a shield when you do speak with him. By being psychically aware, you can put your psychic senses to good use and help you with your everyday life.

You should understand that your psychic senses couldn't help you if you do not make good use of them.

It is noteworthy that the word "psychic" comes from the word psi, which means energy. Hence, when you talk about psychic awareness, it has to do with being aware of the energy inside you and all around you. By sensing and understanding energy, you will be more able to know the best actions to take in any situation. Hence, it can help you come up with the best decision and course of action.

Empathy

The key to psychic awareness is to develop empathy. Empathy is another psychic ability that will allow you to sense human emotions and feelings. Technically speaking, it is not just emotions that you can sense when you develop empathy. Instead, you get to sense and understand energy, especially the quality of energy.

So, how do you develop empathy? Again, you can develop empathy by doing the exercises in this book. There are also certain practices that you can do that directly engage and develop this ability. Let us discuss them one by one:

Empathic connection

The next time that you interact with someone, visualize a cord that connects your heart chakra to the heart chakra of the other person. Keep a clear and open mind. How do you feel about it? Is there any idea or thought that pops into your mind as you connect to this person? Try to sense the state of mind of the other person. When done, do not forget to cut the link. You can do this by visualizing that you are psychically cutting the link with a visualized scissors or knife.

Psychic sense

An easy way to use empathy is simply to be still and just feel the other person. How do you feel about him/her? When you use this technique, you need to clear your mind. Having a clear mind will allow you to get impressions from the other person. Use your intuition and psychic senses to know more and understand the other person.

Heart chakra empowerment

The main chakra that is used for empathy is that heart chakra. Therefore, by developing the heart chakra, the more empathic you can be. There is a simple yet effective way to do this, and that is by charging your heart chakra with energy. Simply visualize that whenever you inhale, you get to draw in energy from the universe and allow this energy to flow and charge up your heart chakra. Let the heart chakra be energized until it is shining brightly in your mind's eye. Do this several times a day, and you will definitely have a powerful heart chakra that you can effectively use for empathy.

Listen to your emotions/feelings

Empathy is all about emotions or feelings. The more that you understand the language of feelings, the more that you will be able to know what certain energy impressions mean. Hence, make it a habit to teach yourself to listen to your feelings. The more that you understand certain feelings, the more that you will understand the language behind them.

There are people who are only in touch with their psychic abilities or senses when they meditate or do something that are related to their spiritual practice. This is wrong, as you cannot really separate your psychic self from who you are even during normal consciousness. Hence, learn to live with your psychic abilities and senses.

How to Develop Your Psychic Abilities

Now, how do you enhance these abilities? Well, just like with any other skill, you simply have to keep on practicing them. When you say practice, it means actually putting it into real application. The best way to practice is to incorporate your psychic abilities in your everyday life.

So, how do you live with psychic abilities? Simply make them a natural part of who you are as a person. After all, there is no good reason for you to hide them. However, it should be noted that you should not boast about your abilities, and you should not use them for evil purposes. Let us now discuss effective ways on how to enhance your psychic abilities by making them a part of your everyday life:

- When you take a bath, do not just clean your physical body, but also make an effort to cleanse all negative energies of your astral body. Visualize that as you clean your physical body, you also clean all negativities and impurities in your soul. See and feel the negative energies being washed away by the water and go in down the drain. Visualize yourself shining brightly.

- If you have time to focus on your breath, then you can cleanse and charge yourself at any time. As you inhale, visualize positive energy entering your body. When you exhale, see and feel the negative energies being released from your body.

- When someone calls you on the phone, take a moment to define who it is. Close your eyes or just focus, listen to your intuition, and then focus on who it is.

- When you are engaged in a conversation, do not just listen to the words that the other person is telling you. You should also connect to them on a deeper level by using your empathic ability. Use whatever technique you may find helpful or necessary.

- Make sure to make time to meditate regularly (every day). Meditation plays a very important role in your spiritual development, especially in the awakening of the Kundalini.

- When you see an interesting object, especially if it is an old object, hold it in your hand, feel it, and allow your intuition to tell you the history of the object. This ability is known as psychometry.

- Start using your intuition. This does not mean that you should no longer use logic or reasons, but you should also pay attention to what your intuition tells you.

- Improve yourself by working on corresponding chakras.

There are many ways to incorporate your practices in your daily life. The problem is that there are people who simply do not take the efforts to practice their abilities. It is also advised that you give yourself even just an hour from time to time to do nothing but to practice your abilities. You do not have to develop all your psychic abilities all at once. If you want, you can just focus on one or two abilities at a time.

The more that you make good use of your abilities, the more that you can develop them. The key here is repetition. This is why continuous practice is very important. You also have to give it your focus and attention. Always do your best.

Chapter 5: Psychic Skills

This is another great topic in spirituality. When you practice the techniques in this book, you are going to wake up your psychic abilities. Unfortunately, quite a few people view psychic abilities as something supernatural that doesn't really exits. The truth of the matter is, psychic abilities are real and takes nothing more than healthy and strong chakras and an open mind. There are several different types of psychic abilities. Let's go over each one.

Clairvoyance

This is the most common ability. Clairvoyance is having an ability of clear-seeing. Clairvoyants are often able to see symbols, dreams, visions, images, and colors that help them to interpret their environment. These images will either be seen with the physical or mind's eye.

Clairvoyance gives you a way to access the knowledge of your own soul, and the collective knowledge of every soul within the Universe. This includes the past, present, and those not yet here. Unfortunately, there are many people who are clairvoyant that discredit this ability as a daydream, imagination, or wishful thinking.

These people aren't completely wrong. Clairvoyance does originate from the same side of the brain as the imagination, the right side. However, the imagination holds the seeds for these clairvoyant images. This is why these images appear in the same way as all other free expression and creativity.

You can tell when your clairvoyance is strengthening when you experience:

- Extremely vivid or active dreams.

- You daydream more than usual.

- You are able to come up with entire scenes about the future within your mind.

- When you are listening to a conversation, you start playing out an inner scene in your mind where you can see it unfold.

- You have a way with descriptive metaphors.

- You start seeing things out of the corner of your eye which causes you to do a double take to make sure that you didn't really see a person.

- You have blurry vision or see flashes of light.

- You experience precognitive visions during meditation or in dreams.

- When you notice a spirit in your space, you feel as if you can see it within your mind and you feel that you know what the spirit looks like.

These all show that you have a sharp inner vision, which, with more work, can be sharpened even further, and the exercises in this section will help you do so. Visualization helps clairvoyance ability, as you will see with these exercises.

This first exercise uses a room in your house to help strengthen your clairvoyance:

- Sit in a relaxing position as if you are getting ready to meditate.

- Think about a specific room in your house. It could be the kitchen, bedroom, whichever one speaks to you.

- See it as clearly as possible. Pay attention to all the small details like how objects are arranged, the walls, ceiling, floor, or anything else. Take mental notes of everything you see.

- Open your eyes and go check to see if you were actually able to see everything in the room you chose.

This exercise allows you to travel and see places through clairvoyance. You can use the visualization screen we talked about earlier. Don't rush this technique. Take the time you need so you can take all the mental notes about every little detail.

This next exercise uses flowers. You can either take a walk through the woods or collect several different types of flowers, or you can go to the craft store and buy some fake flowers. The latter is a good option for the fall or winter, or if you have allergies. Here's what you do:

- Pick up one of the flowers that you collected and run your fingers all over it.

- Take note of all of its imperfections, textures, and colors.

- Once you believe that you have a good mental image of the flower, close your eyes and lay the flower down.

- Take in a deep breath and allow yourself to relax.

- With your eyes shut, try to recall everything you can about the flower that you just studied. Bring a picture of this flower up in your mind's eye.

- Once you have gotten a good mental image of one flower, you can repeat the process with another flower.

In this last exercise, you get to get creative. You will need a lot of craft supplies; vibrant colored paper, glitter, markers, washi tape, paint, whatever you have on hand.

- Grab a piece of paper and draw out your initials and then start to decorate it. Cover your initials in any fashion that you so wish. The more stuff you are able to add, the more you will get from this exercise.

- Once you are finished decorating your initials, sit and stare at your creation for 30 seconds or so.

- Shut your eyes and allow yourself to relax.

- With your eyes shut, try to think of everything that is on your drawing and hold that image in your mind. Move that mental picture around so that you can watch how the glitter sparkles when the light hits it.

- Open your eyes and see how much you remembered about your drawing.

With your first few attempts, you will probably fail to see every single thing correctly but don't let this discourage you. Keep a positive frame of mind and practice. Never let any failure discourage you. You won't ever fail as long as you continue to try. The more you practice, the better you will get at it. This is how the process works. It is the same as learning any new skill. Keep practicing and do the best you can.

With time and patience, you will soon see progress. You will begin to see that you can visualize the place clearly and you will be able to correctly see where specific things are. This power uses the third eye chakra. The more you practice this you will be able to start visiting other dimensions and places. This might seem like a simple exercise but it is very powerful. All of these techniques are simple, but with constant and sincere practice, it can make a huge difference.

These exercises aren't the only way to strengthen your clairvoyance. You can also play some fun games. Do you remember playing the game Memory as a child? To refresh your memory, the game consisted of at least six cards of three pairs. They would be laid face down, and you would flip them over and try to find the pairs. You can use this same game to help improve your intuitive abilities. You can also enlist the help of a friend and a pack of Zener cards. The cards have different symbols on it and you and your friend can take turns trying to guess the symbols on the cards.

Telekinesis

This psychic ability means someone has the ability to influence or move objects with their mind. There are two types of telekinesis: macro telekinesis and micro telekinesis. Macro telekinesis refers to the way many people understand what telekinesis is. Micro telekinesis refers to having the ability to influence odds or randomness. Meaning you could influence a deck of cards that have been shuffled or a random number generator.

The best way to understand what macro and micro telekinesis are is to do an actual practice:

Macro telekinesis

This is what most people visualize when they hear the word telekinesis. It is the ability to move objects with your mind like moving objects such as a car or a television along with small things like rings or coins. Most people wonder if this is a real ability. This would be a big yes. There are no limits to the power of our minds except what we put upon it. This exercise will help you experience macro telekinesis:

Put a light object in front of you on a table.

Focus your entire attention on this object. Become one with it.

Allow your focus to take over you so that you see nothing but that object.

Make a tunnel with your mind that will connect you to that object and don't allow anything but that object to exist.

Feel the object become one with your mind.

With your mind's eye, watch your astral hand reach out and push the object.

Did you move it? A different way to do it is to just use willpower and be one with the object while making it move with sheer willpower. Many people might have to use visualization. Try both ways and figure out which one works best for you. Don't get discouraged if nothing happens when you first try this. You just have to keep practicing.

Here is one more exercise you could try. This exercise teaches you how to levitate an object. Try these steps:

- Put a light object like a feather on your hands.

- Keep your hands with your palms up in front of you.

- Feel the feather on your palms. Feel its weight. Its lightness.

- You are going to use your energy to levitate this feather. You are going to draw energy by chanting: "light as air, light as a feather."

- Continue chanting this for a few minutes while you connect with the object and cause it to levitate.

If you don't have a feather, you could use aluminum foil. The foil might not levitate, but it might move a bit on your hand.

Macro telekinesis is thought of as an advanced psychic ability. Don't expect to have the ability to do these exercises without taking time to practice them for a long time. This ability is worth learning. Don't let it cause you to lose sight of what is most important in your spiritual life. Acquiring psychic powers is interesting and nice, but it isn't the end all be all of your spirituality.

Micro telekinesis

You will need a coin to do this exercise. Remember micro telekinesis is influencing the outcome of odds or randomness. For this exercise, you are going to use your mind to change the outcome of the flip of a coin. Any coin will do as long as it has two different sides. Now you need to pick either heads or tails. You are going to influence your side so that it will land up with each flip of the coin. You must influence this coin while flipping it 100 times.

In theory, if you flip a coin 100 times, the outcome would normally be 50 tails and 50 heads or something close to that. If you are able to apply micro telekinesis, then you should have a large difference such as 70 tails and 30 heads, if tails were your chosen side.

How can you do this? How can you apply micro telekinesis? The best way is doing it with your mind and by using visualization and willpower. Here are the steps:

- Relax completely since telekinesis is better when you are completely relaxed.

- You aren't trying to force anything to happen. Instead, you are letting it happen. Let's say your chosen side is tails.

- When you flip the coin, "see" with your mind that the coin will fall with the tail side up.

- While doing this, exert very strong willpower. You are commanding the coin to do your will.

Here is a different technique you could try:

- Choose a coin and put it in your hand.

- Look at it and keep your focus on it. Become one with it. Focus until it feels like it is a part of you.

- When you feel you are in complete control, use your willpower to influence it and make it give you your outcome.

While flipping the coin, feel the coin as being a part of you and make it land on the side you want it to.

There aren't any secrets to this technique. It is just about being one with the coin and making it do your will. Don't think of the coin as being a separate object.

Feel like you are one with the coin or it is an extension of you such as an elbow or leg. You have become that coin.

This is only an example of the way micro telekinesis could be used. If you get to a point where it is easy for you to control the outcome of the coin flip, you could try new things like dice or a deck of cards that has been shuffled. When using a deck of cards, you could try to just force a certain color. Think of either black or red while shuffling the deck. The top card of the deck will be the chosen color. You have free rein on how you practice using micro telekinesis. After you have developed this ability, you can use it in many ways. There are people who claim that they can use this to influence slot machines or the lottery. There are actual psychics who have won the lottery. Understand that psychic abilities aren't meant to be used to make you rich. You need to use them to help others and grow better spiritually. Don't lose the real purpose when practicing these abilities. Remain steadfast in what is good.

Clairsentience

This is known as clear sensing. This lets you feel the future, past, or present along with the emotional states of others without using the normal five senses. With this ability, you can feel any subtle energy. Look at it like this: if clairvoyance is about sight, clairsentience is about feelings. This isn't as hard as it seems. You might already have a good sense of clairsentience and you just aren't aware of it yet. A good example is having a bad feeling right before something bad happens. You might feel positive energy and realize that you had a spirit brush by you. This deals a lot with the quality of energy. How can you practice and develop this ability? Just keep feeling the energy. If you can develop your empathic ability, you will be able to increase your clairsentience. Try this exercise:

1. You need to be in a public place or someplace where there are a lot of people around you.

2. Look around and find someone that you "feel" is a good person. You don't need to be logical here just let your intuition lead you.

3. Discreetly focus on this person.

4. Feel with your heart chakra. Your heart chakra is the center of your emotions. It is Universal oneness and love.

5. Feel and see a ray of light coming from your heart chakra and allow it to connect with your

chosen person's heart chakra. This will be your connection to this person.

6. Clear your mind. You should soon be receiving ideas, thoughts, emotions, or impressions from this person.

You aren't limited to just feeling people's energy. You can use your ability to sense a place's energy. If you don't like or are afraid of traveling, you could think of a place in your mind and try to "feel" it from afar. Like with any other skill, this is also going to take practice. The main point is to use your feelings to sense the energy around you. The more you practice, the more sensitive you will get to all the subtle energy.

Divination

A simple definition of divination is seeking knowledge about the future by using supernatural or unknown means. It comes from the Latin divinare meaning to foresee or being inspired by a god. It is an attempt to get insight about a situation or question by using standardized, occult rituals or processes.

Tarot cards are the most common tool used by people who have this ability. We will not be going in depth about each tarot card, but I will teach you how to use any type of tarot deck. You use your intuition. All tarot cards give you a message that you have to figure out. Rather than every card having a specific meaning, you can also interpret the meanings in your own way. Again you do this by using your intuition.

There aren't any set rules on how to do this. You just need to choose a card or create a spread. When you have the cards in front of you that you have to interpret, just clear your mind and relax. Let your intuition take total control. Look at the cards and focus on them. How are you feeling? Are you getting any emotions or ideas from the cards? Take your time so you can understand each card. When you have practiced enough, you will get better and be able to read all the tarot cards. You have to understand that the tarot cards are mere tools. There aren't any regulations or rules. You are using them to give you a message. It isn't practical to memorize every meaning of every card.

One other method of divination is using pendulums. For doing this, you need to learn to dowse. You might be wondering what a pendulum is. This is an object that has been suspended from a chain or string. Before you can practice this, you need to have a pendulum. You can find them in any occult shop. If you are just beginning, you can create your own. You just need a thread or string and a needle. A normal sewing needle is fine. Just cut the thread to whatever length you desire and place it through the eye of the needle and tie it off.

When you use dowsing, pendulums can answer your questions. The best questions are ones that can be answered by either no or yes. You can ask it a question like: "Will it rain today?" It will then swing in the direction that you have dictated to be "yes" or "no". A pendulum is a very effective tool when used correctly. Now that you have a general idea about using a pendulum, let's try a little exercise.

You need to find out how your pendulum will move for a "yes" or "no" answer. You can figure this out be holding your pendulum by the string and let it hang freely. When it becomes still, ask it to show you "yes". The pendulum should move in a specific direction. This will indicate how it will answer for "yes". Remember how it moved. Now do the same thing for "no". Don't stop until you understand how it is going to respond for you. You should have two very distinctive motions for the answer of "yes" and "no". When you have your responses, you can begin asking questions.

Don't try to ask hard questions when starting out. You need to warm up and get used to your pendulum. Your first questions need to be ones that you know the answer to already like: "Am I wearing black pants?" or "Is today Tuesday?" See if the pendulum gives you the right response. When you are used to this, then you can use it to answer questions that you don't know the answer to. Let's begin:

1. Let the pendulum hang freely while holding onto the end of the chain or string.

2. Allow the "needle" to hang freely and allow it to get still. When it stops moving, ask your question.

3. Make sure you ask your question the right way meaning that is can only be answered by either a yes or no answer. Keep the question clear and short.

4. When asking your questions, be completely focused on it.

5. If it doesn't give you a clear answer, repeat these question until it begins to move.

6. You can ask your pendulum any number of questions you would like to, just remember to ask them in the correct way.

Dowsing is a skill just like any other and it requires practice. Never expect to get the correct answers when you are just learning. You have to practice, practice, and practice some more. You should only use one pendulum in order to create a good connection with it. If you need to cleanse your pendulum of negative energies, you can wash it under running water or by submerging it into salt water for a few seconds. You could also put it outside and let the rain cleanse it. Dowsing is an interesting practice. It can be used to find missing people, hidden treasures, lost objects, or water. It can also give you answers to your biggest questions.

Psi Healing

This is the ability to heal by using prana. This is an ability that can be learned. You will learn how to heal illnesses and ailments with prana. There are several ways you can do this. You could find a school for pranic or Reiki healing and take classes. Both use prana to heal but there are some differences. Reiki uses symbols whereas prana focuses on energy healing without actually touching. Let's look at an exercise that will help you understand it better:

- You might have a part of you that doesn't feel well. Let's say it is your knee. You can fill it with prana to help heal it. You do this by charging your knee with energy.

- Inhale and visualize your knee absorbing pranic energy. Feel that energy going deep into your knee.

- Continue doing this until it is completely full of prana.

- You need to make sure you have true intentions and faith to heal by using prana.

Our bodies were made to heal themselves. We have forgotten how to do this because today's practices have blocked our bodies from using its healing powers. When we charge the affected part with prana, you are helping it to heal. Remember when healing it will take a lot of energy. You could try this technique any time you have a stomach ache, headache, toothache, or wherever you might have pain. If you were to develop a fever, you can charge your entire body with prana.

When you get good at this, you could use the ability to heal others. Healing with energy is one of the many abilities that everyone seems to want to learn. Remember that as with all abilities, this is within your grasp to learn. It also takes a lot of practice, especially meditation.

There are numerous psychic abilities in the world. There are just too many to name. All of these use the exact same energy. It is how the energy gets used that makes them different. Acquiring psychic abilities is a part of the spiritual path but it isn't the end that you are looking for.

Many traditions reject psychic abilities because people thought they would get in the way of attaining true enlightenment. This all depends on a person's preference or beliefs and in how you use these abilities. You need to learn how to use your abilities properly and help people in any way possible for the good.

Awareness

Psychic awareness will happen when you learn how to use your chakras. When you are becoming more psychic, you are becoming more aware of energy or prana within you. Remember everything has energy. When you do the techniques in this book, you will become more sensitive to energy. This will enhance and increase your psychic awareness.

To become more aware, you need to work on intuition. Basically, you need to make sure your third eye is open. Think about seeing your physical things by using your normal eyes, you can use your third eye to see the energy around you. You can use other senses, too.

Awareness is one thing, understanding is another. You need to be careful with this. Some practitioners learn how to be aware but don't do anything else. If you don't do anything, this you really aren't aware of anything. This happens when people don't trust their intuition. If you feel danger when going into a certain place, you need to leave that place immediately. Don't wait until something bad happens. Trust your intuition. When you don't trust your psychic awareness, you will begin to lose it. Some believed all humans had strong psychic awareness. Parents began training their children to focus on physical objects and we forgot about our natural abilities to be aware of energy around us as we grew up. This should have never happened. You need to remember your psychic senses and begin learning how to use them again.

Enhancement

Is there a way to enhance psychic abilities? The simple answer is practice. When you practice, you will continue to get better. This is the main reason people don't succeed in life. Constant practice isn't easy. Many people stop halfway and abandon whatever it is they are doing. When learning new skills, it requires a lot of practice. Let's say you want to learn how to play the piano. You are given a book with clear instructions on how and where to place your fingers along with where each key is located. You are not going to be perfect on your first couple of tries. It might even take you weeks to be able to play through an entire song without making a mistake.

This same thing happens when you are learning how to achieve any psychic ability. Knowing how to do it is important but it isn't enough. The other important element is to constantly practice. These are the two elements for success: the correct knowledge and constant practice. This book gives you the knowledge. You have to turn that knowledge into practice.

Here are some steps that will help you enhance your psychic abilities:

Believe in yourself

Having negative thoughts can hinder your psychic abilities. You have to have faith and remain positive. Find inspiration anytime, anyplace, and anywhere. Read about other people who have developed their psychic abilities and learn how they did it. Release all skepticism. Trust your natural power along with the supernatural powers in the world. If you give anything less than 100 percent, it isn't acceptable. There isn't any room for doubt while on a spiritual journey.

Relax

In order to get into deep relaxation, many people will breathe slowly or meditate while thinking about nothing. It will clear your mind but it also changes the patterns of the brain waves. It can also relieve tension and decrease metabolic rate. It could improve heart health and cure hypertension. Meditation temporarily alters the prefrontal cortex. This lets your brain perform better and boosts your energy levels. This is what you need to do to get in touch with your spiritual self. Release all your stress and breathe.

Take care of problems

You can't be in tune with your psychic gifts if you aren't at peace with the people around you and yourself. Stay away from fighting. If an argument happens, be quick to resolve it. When you argue, always work toward a resolution. Trying to hurt everyone while angry will make the problem worse. It is harder to meditate when you have a lot of weight on your shoulders. You will never be able to clear your head.

Overcome fears

Psychic abilities can be a bit frightening but being afraid of them will keep your abilities at bay more than being negative. If you truly want to be in tune with your spiritual side, you can't be scared of any consequences. You might get a vision when you least expect it. This is all part of the experience. Embrace your gift. Think of the good you could do with this power and you might not be so scared.

Stay positive

Do what you need to do to stay positive in life. This might entail taking time each day just to do something for yourself. Find a hobby that you like to do. Just find something to put a smile on your face. Negativity and stress will keep you from being completely relaxed. You have to feel free spiritually to be able to improve your psychic abilities. Release your worries before trying to get into a deep state of consciousness.

Improve psychometry skills by finding objects with unknown histories

When you have found objects with unknown histories, touch them until you begin to get feelings. Try to connect to their past. Concentrate for however long it takes. Can you feel anything about its history, its owners, or the item itself? Never force any visions. Just hold the item and feel your way. Don't put any pressure on yourself. Don't get frustrated if you don't feel anything. This will happen from time to time. Every object isn't going to have a past.

Increase telepathy by reading other's thoughts

You have the ability to communicate with others silently. You can practice by guessing what others are thinking whenever possible. Have a person draw a picture or select a card from a deck. Try to figure out what they are drawing or what card was drawn without getting any clues. Continue doing this daily. Telepathy takes concentration and could take years to completely develop. It will get easier with practice and time.

Chapter 6: Clairvoyance & Other Psychic Gifts

If you approached kundalini awakening in the first place hoping for some level of psychic awakening, don't feel dejected or misled. Kundalini awakening will absolutely align you better with your intuition, deeper insights, and soul's mission. Furthermore, it will allow you to unlock additional psychic gifts on levels you may not have even known existed before your kundalini rose. This section will walk you through several different psychic gifts that are possible to attain, and as you strengthen your general manifestation and attraction abilities with kundalini awakening, you may even be able to pick and choose these gifts for your experience and needs, based on what you read below.

Aura reading is another psychic gift that is basically exactly what it sounds like. Many of us have the gift of aura reading in our own way, and if anyone tries to tell you that only *one* version of aura reading is right, they're not telling you the full truth. Everyone who can see auras sees them a little bit differently because everyone is unique in their own way. Therefore, if you believe you can see auras, but it doesn't fit with others' experiences, don't worry; trust yourself and believe in your gift.

Automatic writing is a psychic gift that involves channeling (the next point in this list) to a certain extent. Essentially, this gift allows the writer to be able to channel his or her higher self, guides, angels, guardians, or more in that person's effort to be verbally creative.

Channeling is a psychic gift that allows the individual to enter a trance and let another spirit speak through them for a time. It's sort of like demonic or angelic possession, but it's voluntary. The person who acts as the channel will almost always be fully willing to let the spirit talk through him or her.

Clairaudience is a psychic gift that revolves around the ability to hear outside the standard range of human hearing. People with these gifts would be able to hear into other planes of existence, even into supernatural worlds.

Clairgustance is an unusual psychic gift that is oriented around taste and eating. Individuals with this gift would randomly get a taste in their mouth and then receive messages later on in relation to that taste. Furthermore, these "clear tasters" would be able to taste something before even putting it on their tongue.

Clairsalliance is a psychic gift that revolves around the ability to smell outside the standard range of human smelling. Perhaps you would smell something before it happened (such as spilled food or a gas main break or fire). Perhaps you would be able to smell someone's vice on him or her before even striking up conversation. The possibilities are virtually endless!

Clairsentience is the psychic gift that allows one to simply feel the presence of something more. Whether that "more" is a spirit, a guide, an ancestor, a demon, or what have you, this individual would sense the physical (or spiritual) energy of that being before anyone else.

Clairvoyance is a more commonly-heard-of psychic gift that features the ability to see information in one's mind. These people might receive visions or see physical insights into others' lives, but the gist is the same each time: things are always visual.

Divination is the general application of one's psychic gifts to find answers to questions. Divination can be used in terms of reading palms, tea leaves, I Ching, natal charts, tarot cards, crystals, runes, and so much more.

Dowsing is a more old-school psychic gift that our ancestors used to find things. Sometimes, dowsing is guided with a rod or sticks, but the point is to find what's important to you (it was often water or shelter) when you might even have no idea what you're looking for.

Empathy is a psychic gift that allows you to literally feel or take on the emotions of another person. Empaths are often highly sensitive to the feelings of others to a detrimental degree until they learn how to ground themselves and protect their energy from all-too-natural invasion by others.

Intuition is an underrated psychic gift, for it truly is an example of precognition. Anyone whose intuition was right essentially received a momentary glimpse into the future, so the next time *your* intuition is right, be proud for you're unlocking psychic gifts as you live and breathe! There's the first piece of proof!

Mediumship is the highly-coveted psychic ability of contacting those who have passed. Many people are fascinated (if not obsessed) with communing with the spirits of those who are no longer living, and kundalini awakening can help you get there, but you'll really want to be careful. Mediumship can be an incredibly draining gift, and it's not for the faint of heart. I guess what I'm saying is this: be careful what you wish for.

Premonition is the psychic ability of being able to see into the future. This gift is often more symbolic than literal, but the gist is the same whether the message is literal or figurative: the individual with the gift of premonition will know of future events before they come to pass.

Psychometry is a sense-based psychic gift that connects the individual with truth or facts about an object, thing, animal, place, or person just by touching it.

Retrocognition is the psychic ability of being able to see into the past with varying degrees of detail. Sometimes, those glimpses are into one's past lives, while other times, they're general peeks into the past that have no relation to your experience (as far as you know!).

Telekinesis is a psychic ability that allows the individual to manipulate matter with his or her mind, whether moving it, energizing it, or otherwise. Telekinetic individuals can sometimes do such amazing things as walk through walls, bend firm objects, trash a room without being in it, call people to their aid without speaking, and more.

Telepathy is the final psychic gift we'll discuss, and it relates to the power of the individual to communicate with others without opening one's mouth. This alternative mode of communication would likely be through thought, emotion, or vibration.

Chapter 7: Astral Travel

Astral travel is something that most people find a mystery, but it is something that has grown in popularity. While a lot of people still find it odd, it's important to know that you and everybody else do astral travel every time you sleep. Very few people are able to remember what happens when they travel.

Astral travel, for those who don't know, is where your astral body leaves your physical body and travels to some other area. This is an interesting thing and is a skill that will allow you to travel anywhere in the world without having to pay. You can see the Great Wall, the Taj Mahal, Ireland, Australia, and any other place you could imagine. You can even visit other magical planes of existence and celestial spheres. This is the main reason why so many people want to learn how to astral travel.

When the subject of astral travel comes up, something a lot of people will ask is how safe it is. This is a fair question. Astral travel is the separation of the physical and astral body, but death is really nothing more than a permanent separation of the two bodies, so that means it must be dangerous, right? Not exactly. Astral travel is actually very safe. You don't have to be afraid of it because you have already been doing it for years. The only difference is that you weren't aware of it. Learning to astral travel will allow you to do so and remember your trips.

Fear is very common when it comes to learning about astral travel. I can tell you a million times that it is safe, but it's not easy to believe what I say. How can it not be scary when you notice that you are no longer a part of your physical body? Practice is what will help you to work through this fear. Fear is one of the main reasons why astral travel doesn't work for some people. Fear will cause you to pull your astral body back into your physical body. This is why it's important that you learn how to conquer this fear. You have to understand that this is completely safe.

As soon as you feel afraid, even if just the slightest bit, you will be yanked back into your physical body. Returning to your physical body is extremely easy to do. All you have to do is will yourself back. Simply thinking, "I want to be back in my body," is enough to take you to it. This is why you need to have good control over your thoughts. The important thing is that you cultivate a positive mindset and try not to be afraid. Furthermore, a negative mindset while astral traveling will cause you to attract negative entities.

Again, you don't need to worry about these things because you will be brought back to your physical body before you face any actual danger.

While astral traveling, some people experience the silver cord. This silver cord is like an umbilical cord that connects your astral and physical body. This shows you that your two bodies are never really separated. Not everybody witnesses this silver cord. If you don't see one, that is not a big deal. If you do see one, don't worry about it; continue on with your journey.

When you travel, you may see your physical body and possibly your astral form, but you could also appear as nothing but consciousness. You might see the things around you or you could just hear. The more you practice this skill, the better you will become.

You may even encounter other entities or beings in the astral plane. When you are first starting out, it is best that you try not to communicate with anyone or anything in the astral world. As long as you ignore them, they won't bother you. Again, there is no need to be afraid. If you start to sense danger, you can head back to your physical body. If something bad starts to happen, your astral body will automatically be pulled back into your body.

Not only will you be able to travel to amazing places with this, but will also help you to deal with any fears you have concerning death. Death is only the permanent separation of your physical and astral body. With astral travel, it's only temporarily. This will serve as proof that there is life after your physical body perishes.

Most people want to learn astral travel because of its wonderful benefits. The great thing is that everybody has the ability to learn how. Like with any other ability or skill, you have to practice. Luckily, you sleep every night, so practice is easy. With astral travel, the body sleeps, but your consciousness stays awake. We're going to go through some different methods of travel.

Travel Methods

Mental Travel: This isn't technically astral traveling, but it is a good place for people to start. Once you have become skilled in this, it will help you to get into real astral traveling. This will only need you to use your mind. Your astral and physical bodies will start together. Depending on how powerful your visualization skills are, this could become an astral journey for you. Follow these steps.

1. Get into a comfortable position, laying down. Allow yourself to relax. Take a deep breath in and out and relax as if you are going to sleep. Make sure that you stay awake mentally and that your spine remains straight.

2. Visualize the room that you are in. Use your mental eyes to see through your closed eyes. Do your best to look all around your room and pay close attention to the small details and the objects you have in your room.

3. Visualize yourself stepping out of this room and into the next room of your house. Visualize this room clearly, like you did the first. Continue to move through the rooms of your house as if you were walking to your front door.

4. Step outside of your house and then roam about your neighborhood and travel wherever you want.

5. Once you are finished with your travels, all you need to do is to visualize the room that you are in and think about your physical body. Slowly start to wiggle your toes and fingers and then open your eyes.

This may be nothing but a visualization exercise; it is also helpful to get your mind ready. When you do this, make sure that you visualize these places as clearly as you can. This isn't astral traveling because you won't have to visualize when you travel, but this is still a great step in the right direction.

Roll-Out Method: In this method of astral traveling, you separate your two bodies by rolling onto your side.

1. Lay down and get ready to go to sleep. Your body is going to fall asleep, but your consciousness will be awake. Lay there and allow your body to relax, rest, and sleep.

2. As you do this, feel and think that you are just an astral being. Keep this mindset for a few minutes. When you feel that you have become connected with your astral body, believing that you are your astral body and not a physical

one, you should notice that the physical being is asleep, but your astral body remains conscious.

3. After you have reached this, you will roll out to the side and leave your astral body. If everything goes well, you will notice that you are no longer a part of your physical body and that you are your astral body.

4. Make sure that you don't allow fear to creep in. It can be startling to see your physical body sleeping there in front of you, but if you allow yourself to become afraid, you will be pulled back into your physical body.

5. You should only roll over onto your side once you no longer feel connected with your physical body. This may have to be tried several times so that you can learn the right sensation or signal for the rolling motion. You can roll to either side that you want; the important thing is to do this with your astral body.

Floating: This one will have you float out of your physical body.

1. As always, lay down and become relaxed. Your spine needs to be straight. Take a deep breath in and out and allow yourself to relax, but don't fall asleep. Your physical body should be the only thing that falls asleep.

2. Feel yourself in your astral body and not your physical body. Look around your room with just your astral eyes. Let the physical body to continue to relax and fall asleep.

3. Notice that when you inhale, your astral being will become lighter. As you feel lighter, you will begin to float. You will first float above your physical body, and then you will float higher.

4. At this point, stop thinking about your breath. Focus on the feel of your astral body. Identify with only your astral body and continue to float higher. Move so that you above your house and floating in the clouds.

5. What kinds of things do you see? You have now made it into the astral. Now, all you have to do is think of a place you want to travel to. Think about that place and you will instantly be transported there. If you don't have a particular place in mind, you can simply roam around your neighborhood.

6. Once you want to return home, think about your bedroom. When you are back in your room, watch your physical body sleep. Move closer and enter it. Wiggle your toes and fingers and slowly open your eyes.

Third Eye: With this technique, you will need an open third eye. Through your third eye, you will separate your two bodies.

1. Lay down and relax. As your physical body falls asleep, your mind remains awake. Your spine should be straight so that your energy flow is not interrupted.

2. Once you are feeling relaxed, start to focus on being only your astral body. Notice how you feel trapped inside of your physical body. Picture the glowing indigo light of your third eye and see it as a gateway. This is going to lead you into the astral.

3. Focus on your chakra and view it as a way to enter the astral realm. Move your astral body and leave your physical body through your third eye chakra.

4. Make sure you don't allow yourself to become afraid of seeing your physical body laying there. The third eye chakra is the chakra that is the closest to the spirit world, so it is a great doorway into the astral realm.

All of these techniques can be used for astral travel. Pick the one that you find the easiest to do. There is no need to know how to use all of the techniques perfectly because you only need to use one each time. You can also adjust these techniques as well. There aren't any specific rules that you have to follow for astral travel. Most of the time, astral traveling will happen unintentionally where you become conscious of it once you have left your physical body. These techniques are helpful because you can intentionally travel and choose exactly where you want to go.

Helpful Hints

There are a few different things you can do to help make you more successful when you try to astral travel.

Relax

You won't be able to astral travel when you aren't relaxed. The less relaxed you are, the more attached you are to your physical body. It's important that you make sure your body is so relaxed that it is asleep and that your mind stays focused. When you start out, don't try to think of it as astral traveling. Try to focus on getting your body relaxed like you were just going to sleep.

Have an empty stomach

It is best to astral travel when you have an empty stomach. If you are full, your energy will be divided because your body needs the energy to digest your food, so make sure you don't try this right after you have eaten. Make sure it has been at least two hours since you ate before you try astral traveling. A light snack is fine, but not a large meal. You need your energy for your travels.

Practice regularly

Just like with anything, it's important that you practice regularly. It's a good idea to practice this every night before you go to sleep. If you tend to always fall asleep and lose consciousness, then you may want to try this early each morning. Your body will already be rested and you will be less likely to fall asleep.

Don't expect anything

Expectations tend to ruin astral travel. Release your expectations. You shouldn't even expect to be successful. Expecting something will take away the energy that you need for your travels. It can also end up adding pressure, which isn't going to help you. Instead, try to really relax. While you may know what to expect when you do this, it is a better idea to forget all of this when you start your induction. Focus on what you need to do and forget everything else.

Psychic protection

This is not a requirement, but it's good to help alleviate any fear you may have and to add some extra protection. The following are some good ways to protect yourself.

Remove negative thoughts when traveling.

Sprinkle some saltwater on yourself before you start your travels. This will protect you from negative energies.

Place a circle of salt around your bed.

Picture a white ball of light around your body. This is shielding you of negative energies.

Say a quick prayer before your travel, asking for protection.

Put a cup of salt water next to your body or on a table nearby. Saltwater cleanses and repels negative energies.

Chapter 8: How to awaken kundalini

Most strategies and activities are said to help you improve your well-being or reach your personal fulfillment. This makes it difficult to know what works for you really and what is deceptive or literally useless. However, a search of self-help literature shows hundreds of unfamiliar words, so that you can quickly shrug and move on. You have to remove your prana (or life force) from its constant emphasis on external world awareness if you want to awake your Kundalini. You need to find ways to isolate your senses from what's going on in your physical body because you can only reach the Kundalini's potent energy. As you may already learn from mindfulness or meditation, it can be difficult even for a moment to make such a change, no matter for long periods of time. But even a moment of success will start to shift your thoughts and focus! Through reality, the prana can become second nature in the right way. The good news is that there are small changes you make to wake up your Kundalini.

Here are some of the most powerful methods.

Focus On Your Breath

Anything that makes you focus on your breath allows you also to wake up to Kundalini. This means you are well on the path to tap into your Kundalini energies if you already have a daily meditation or awareness of the kind described above. Don't panic, though, if you are just beginning to figure out such strategies! After all, the shortest types are often the strongest. For starters, try focusing on deep breathing for just five minutes. Inhale through your nose and exhale through your chin, rather than through your lungs. Yoga (not only Kundalini yoga) is another wonderful meditation practice. Whether you are an expert or a new beginner, it can be useful to focus on yoga poses at the beginning of the end of the day. And just remember that you don't have to spend too much time on these exercises to change things.

Reject Negativity

Because you know even if you follow the law of attraction and manifestation, positivity is essential to achieving happiness. In fact, if you want to awaken the Kundalini, you must consciously resist negativity. Most of us are limited to unproductive thought patterns. However, you are slowly developing new patterns by making a concerted attempt to develop a different way of viewing the world. Reframing is one of the best techniques to resist criticism. Whenever you talk about yourself or the world around you, encourage yourself to reword it more positively. "It is far too cold for a sprint today," for instance, "I have the whole afternoon to spend anything I want indoors." Something like "I didn't get the job because I am worthless" becomes more dramatic: "I haven't got this job because the right one comes in the corner."

Keep A Good Posture

There is a very close relationship between the physical body and the Kundalini awakening. It is particularly important to keep an eye on your posture and make changes when appropriate. If you have a fairly sedentary job that takes long hours on a screen, like most men, you may be likely to hunch with round shoulders. Likewise, fatigue can leave you with tight muscles, and low self-confidence will intentionally may your body. The most important thing you have to do is keep your back straight so that your back is long and tall. This not only allows you to wake up the kundalini but also strengthens the entire body, reducing chronic pain issues. When it's hard for you to first think about your posture, try to straighten your back a daily reminder. After a week or two, you will no longer need a reminder.

Access The Central Channel

You may not have learned before about the central point, but be certain that the measures to access it are relatively straightforward. Next, make sure you relax and breathe deeply while you are eight. Then concentrate on your tailbone until you feel a soft vibration. Close your eyes at this point and constantly sing the word "Vum." When you sing, remember the sound of vibration slowly up your spine. Adjust your singing, repeat the phrase "shum" over and over while you hear the waves travel across your muscles to fill the entire body and fill the whole body. Imagine a big bubble in your pelvic and abdominal region and fill it. Lets the air out of the ball slowly as if you keep it by the neck and softly remember everything within. More complex activities are given to reach the core channel, but the process begins. Hypnosis might also help you reach your main net! Self-hypnosis will help you relax, concentrate, and awaken your kundalini energies beneath your spine. Seek inner peace and take control of your wellbeing with this hypnosis kundalini.

Use Visualization

Visualization techniques are powerful tools in all life fields and are also necessary if the Kundalini is to be awoken. In particular, when you look at Kundalini Yoga resources, you can find a recurring pattern of light visualizations. The Divine Light Invocation is one of the most common and significant, and it is simple to do, even if you're a novice. Start standing as straight as you can, stretching your feet to about the width of your shoulder. Next, close your eyes slowly and lift them up so that they face to the middle of your lower forehead. When you do, raise your arms and keep all your muscles close above your head. Say this, imagine yourself being bathed in bright white light:

"Divine light makes me. God's love upholds me. Divine light surrounds me and encircles me. I'm rising into divine light all the time.

Activate Your Interests

While working on your role, it is not sufficient just to promote a Kundalini awakening to trigger your interests. It is also important to live a healthy, balanced life! Yet to get the strength of Kundalini inside you, it is important that you spend at least an hour a day on something you really enjoy. You may find it hard to overcome the burden of a society that says that you should spend any minute on productive activity, but participation is beneficial in your interests. What if you don't know where your interests lie anymore? Try listing 10-15 stuff you have wished to do, without any censorship. At least one thing you should start to learn, try, or focus on today is one of these. And if you don't think an attraction satisfying you anymore, just leave it without regret. A good life is important for your Kundalini's awakening.

Cut Out Distractions

Ultimately, we all spend our days of easily frustrating stuff. Our attention is drawn in hundreds of different directions at once, and for very long periods, we can find it hard to concentrate on one thing. But when we allow our minds to shift constantly, we focus externally in a way that refuses us proper access to our

Kundalini's resources. Know, a new disengagement from external things is needed to create room for a new kind of thought and feeling to emerge. To combat distractions, you have to take a hard look at your living room and activities in order to see what you can do without. Make your home and work smoother.

These forms can also contribute to making progress in your Kundalini practice:

Refine your diet: You're what you eat. If you want to awaken your limitless internal energy, use whole, balanced, and plant-based foods to help you exercise. It is important and can help you to decide your thought, mood, and overall health.

Move your body: Care and devotion are required to unlock your energy. This should be the same kind of love come from your body? Make sure that you push your body by exercise, whether it's a long walk, a sequence of stretches, or a fun team sport every day.

Be The Watcher: It seems like it's all going wrong these days. This is something that everybody feels. Rather than getting covered in negative emotions, identify and encourage their presence to pass. You will be happier (emotionally) and more able to concentrate on your Kundalini work.

Find Your Tribe: You subconsciously reflect the people and the environments around you. Choose to engage yourself in only the kindest, most helpful, honest, and most demanding men. Your quality of life will certainly improve when you get good energy.

Get a mentor: Whether it is a fellow yogi or a wise soul, consider someone with whom you can connect deeper. You might even want to share with them your Kundalini experience.

Chant, Chant, Chant: This may be uncommon for yogis practicing in silence, but chanting is a devotional ritual that makes the mood of Kundalini simpler. Find an instructor or something you feel confident practicing to see how chanting helps to make the practice happen.

Enable your interests: We dwell on things several times, and it is not because we enjoy them that we like them. Set aside an hour a day for activities that you feel connected to, be it painting, music, gardening, sports, or programming. Consider whatever it is that you have regular enjoyment.

Here and Now: As you go all day, please make an effort to be mindful of the present moment. Try to cut out international thoughts and focus on the task and the moment. Carefulness also allows you to practice Kundalini and can make you feel relaxed and rooted.

Go with The Flow: Micro-managing your life may seem attractive, but the constant preparation of daily life has liberation. See every morning as an experience you are ready to take part in. Don't freak out if the way you've planned your day doesn't go.

Affirmations: if you can be polite to all around you... but you, your kundalini practice (and your general health and happiness) will collapse. Take your time every day to remember your various strengths, gifts, and virtues.

Listen to music for your relaxation: listening to music or movements that calm your mind and body encourages a meditative state that can help you practice Kundalini. Music helps you to relax and tap into an intrinsic release of energy more easily.

Finally, think of unplugging from the internet every now and then or at least set up a browser extension which restricts your time on websites that encourage delays!

Chapter 9: Terminologies

Kundalini – The Kundalini is located at the base of the spine. It is also referred to *as shakti*. It is the primal force. It is coiled like a serpent. However, it is not made of gross material matter, but of fine energy. Once it is awakened, it rises up through the chakras. It is reported to awaken and develop psychic abilities, as well as the feeling of bliss. Many spiritual gurus consider it a step towards enlightenment. Be careful with the power that awakening the Kundalini brings as you might become too focused on the powers that you miss your objective to attain a higher level of spirituality (enlightenment).

Chakras – Chakras are the energy centers of the body. Seven main chakras run along the spine. This is why when you meditate, it is advised that you keep your spine straight. This is to ensure the free flow of energy through the chakras. Chakras, also known as spinning wheels, act as the vital organs of the spiritual body. It is important to keep the chakras healthy if you want the physical body to be healthy.

Aura – The aura is an energy field that surrounds people, animals, plants, as well as objects. The color and shape of the aura reflect the state of mind and health of the subject. It is also worth noting that before illnesses manifest in the physical plane, they first appear in one's aura.

Astral travel – Astral travel is when the astral body goes on a journey. Astral travel, also known as astral projection, is more common than you might think. Every night, when a person sleeps, they astral travel. The problem is that most people are not aware of what happens on their astral journey. When you learn to do astral travel, you train yourself to astral project conscious consciously. You also get to control what happens on your journey.

Prana – Prana is the all-pervading energy that exists everywhere. It is inside you and all around you. Some people even think that prana is God. It is worth noting that with the right knowledge, prana can be used for various purposes, such as for healing and empowerment.

Third eye – The third eye refers to the ajna chakra. It is the chakra that is located between the eyebrows. This chakra is the seat of intuition and is the key to the power of clairvoyance.

Clairvoyance – This refers to the psychic ability of clear seeing. It refers to the ability to see beyond what the physical eyes can perceive.

Meditation – Meditation depends on the meaning that you give it. Some people see it merely as a way to de-stress. However, it should be noted that in awakening the Kundalini, as well as in achieving enlightenment, the practice of meditation is considered a *must*.

Chi – The term, chi, is the Chinese term for prana. It is the same as prana or energy.

Soft focus – Soft focus is often used as a way to see the aura. It is when you look at something using your peripheral vision.

Dry fasting – Dry fasting is fasting from solid foods and liquid, including water. When you go on a dry fast, you literally do not eat or drink anything at all.

Mind's eye – The mind's eye or inner eye refers to what you see or visualize. It also refers to what you may perceive using your intuition. Many of the practices in this book require you to visualize something in your mind's eye.

Psychic awareness – Psychic awareness refers to how aware you are off energies, as well as other psychic entities and influences. A common result of engaging in regular meditation is having increased psychic awareness.

Telekinesis – It refers to the ability to move objects using the power of the mind. It is divided into two: microkinesis and macrokinesis. Microkinesis refers to the ability to influence the outcome of random generators or random odds, such as a roll of a die or coin flip. Microkinesis is how most people understand what telekinesis is, and that is actually moving objects with the mind.

Pyrokinesis – This is another kinesis ability and it refers to the peer to control fire. Hence, the term, pyro, which means fire.

Divination – Divination refers to the ability to predict the future. It is usually associated with the power of clairvoyance.

Pendulum – A pendulum refers to a weighted object that is suspended on a string or chain. It is normally used for divination.

Conclusion

Thank you for making it through to the end of Kundalini Awakening, let's hope it was informative and able to provide you with all of the tools you need to achieve your goals whatever they may be.

The next step is to continue your practice and see where your path leads. The exercises in this book are rooted in an ancient and mysterious past of Indian culture. They literally could be practiced for years without finding an end. Even the simplest meditation exercise can be practiced for decades without losing its potency and power. This shows the immense amount of potential that humans have to transform their lives and empower themselves that these practices have to offer.

The next step is to reaffirm every day that you are on your way to becoming a better, fuller you. Believe in yourself and your ability to make the changes necessary to realize your goals. Once you've removed the clutter from your mind, you will turn overthinking into focused achieving, each and every day. You may have heard many times over, "easier said than done." Well, you should be excited to learn how to do what you set your mind to do. You've wanted to make a change for a long time. Taking the steps to make your goals come to fruition is something many people never achieve.

It is times like this, after having taken a big step forward in my life, when I begin to reflect on how far I've come. It is hard to appreciate your progress sometimes when you are in the heat of battle and struggling every day during the beginning, middle, or even near the end of your efforts. There is nothing better than stepping up onto that final rung and looking down to see all of those completed steps in your wake.

Remember when you were sitting at square one, unable to free yourself from the chains of overthinking? I know it well—I've been there myself. It takes a great deal of courage to stand up and say, I'm ready to make a change. It saddens me to think that many people continue to overthink and overanalyze throughout their entire lives, missing out on the experiences and appreciation that a free mind can realize. It is easy to slip into the comfortable habits of mindless eating, checking a phone or tablet every few minutes, and going to bed later and later until your system is all out of sorts. Sometimes, it seems too easy to give in and let what's easy overshadow what's worth working for. You don't have to be a slave to overthinking, and maybe it's possible for you to take what you've learned and help change lives around you.

Perhaps you know someone who seems to be struggling with overthinking, stressing out about everyday challenges and stress just like you were at the beginning of your journey. Consider reaching out and sharing what you've learned. Nothing feels better than sharing new knowledge with someone who can use it to make the positive changes you've seen happen in yourself. Maybe it's a coworker, a spouse, or a close friend. Many people from different walks of life will benefit from the changes laid out in this book, so why not share your story!

*By **Spiritual Awakening Academy***

www.ingramcontent.com/pod-product-compliance
Lightning Source LLC
Chambersburg PA
CBHW050732030426
42336CB00012B/1530